LIVING HUMAN

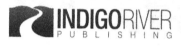

LIVING HUMAN

FLIC MANNING

Indigo River Publishing
3 West Garden Street, Ste. 718
Pensacola, FL 32502
www.indigoriverpublishing.com

Living Human | Flic Manning, author
ISBN: 978-1-950906-59-8 | LCCN: 2020943665

Edited by Adrienne Horn
Cover design by Diesel Laws
Interior design by Robin Vuchnich

Special discounts are available on quantity purchases by corporations, associations, and others. For details, contact the publisher at the address above. Orders by US trade bookstores and wholesalers: Please contact the publisher at the address above.

With Indigo River Publishing, you can always expect great books, strong voices, and meaningful messages.
Most importantly, you'll always find . . . words worth reading.

For Diesel, my "160%," for Grannykins and my family, and for anyone who has struggled. I am with you.

Contents

INTRODUCTION

The definition of *invisible*:

1a: incapable by nature of being seen, or not perceptible
by vision

1b: inaccessible to view, or hidden

2: of such small size or unobtrusive quality as to be hardly
noticeable, or inconspicuous

From around the age of thirteen, I've been put in a box, a category, a
tidy little pigeonhole, called *invisible*, and that is how I have felt for
most of my life. In total juxtaposition to this label or perhaps in some
ways defiance, I've gone on to live a life that's the complete opposite.
On stages in costumes, on music video sets, in fitness studios, founding
a business, and quite often with a microphone thrust into my hands.
And yet *invisible* is the word that still resonates with me at my core.

No, this isn't intended to be a sob story, so please don't put the book
down just yet. Hang in there with me!

I'm a person with a whole life experience. Some of it may be just
like yours. I get up out of bed, I put clothes on, I work, I eat, I watch TV,

I exercise, I have relationships, I sleep (sometimes). But in some ways, my lived experience may differ from yours. And that is partially what I'm here to share.

You see, I face pain and illness a lot. They are close companions of mine. Yet I genuinely love my body. I respect her so much. She fights for me every day, and I for her, and together we have done some pretty awesome things personally and professionally. I'm not special, and as lonely as I have sometimes felt on this journey, I'm never really alone because there are millions of people around the world just like me. I spent years draped in a cloak of shadows and shame which was never mine to have worn in the first place. I am no longer ashamed of my reality. I am no longer hidden in the darkness. I don't remain unseen, unheard, or unnoticed. I refuse to. I'm right here with you as visible as I have ever been.

I'm also a contradiction in terms: *invisible* and *seen*, *introvert* and *extrovert*, a happy soul who carries a lot of trauma inside of her. So I hope that along the way you'll get used to this back-and-forth reality in which I am two sides of the same coin. It is also my hope that this little snapshot of my complex story (as we all have), these lessons that I have learned, often in the most bizarre and trying of ways, serves to help you or someone you know in some way. If not, hopefully, this will be an interesting read digested over a cup of tea, where you can reflect on this thing that you're doing right now, living - having a human experience with all its awesome bits, crap bits, middle-of-the-road bits, painful bits, indescribable bits - and realize that every bit is actually a privilege. Being human, truly human, is an incredible blessing and a super power.

So let's do this. Let's be human together.

WELLNESS TIP:
Meditate

Before you get started, take a moment to meditate.

Please take a deep breath in through your nose and out through your mouth, and keep repeating your breaths in this rhythm. With each exhale, I'd like you to bring your attention to your physical self; relax your body in any way that you are able to, perhaps unclench your jaw, drop your shoulders, soften your gaze, and just let yourself absorb the gravity you feel as it's pulling you down towards the chair, the bed, the floor, the train, the tram, or wherever you may be right now.

After six deep breaths, let go of all of the focus on your breathing and allow your breathing to return to its normal rhythm. When you are ready, gently bring yourself back to the present moment.

Now that you have meditated for a moment and quieted your sympathetic nervous system through the power of your breath, you are ready to begin.

1

THE ORIGIN

Binary opposition: a system of language in which two theoretical opposites are set off or defined against each other. Life, to me, is much the same. I know good because I have known bad. I embrace joy because I have been hugged (read: practically strangled) by despair. I believe that for you to know why I move forward, why I am propelled instead of stagnant, you must know what once held me back. So let's get the dark, icky root of my story out of the way, shall we?!

Let me take you back a couple of decades.

I'm just barely a teen, and for a long time I've been feeling truly and utterly sick. I am permanently nauseated and exhausted and the pain I am in seems to intensify daily. I don't understand what's going on with my body, and I'm now terrified of it. *I'm actually terrified of my own body.* Back when she let me dance (which I love) and act and do karate and play musical instruments and go to school uninterrupted, I really didn't pay her much attention. I just thought she was normal, and we had a good relationship. But now, she and I are at total loggerheads.

I've been poked and prodded for months. I've been spending time in doctors' offices pooping in cups (honestly, why are those cups so small?), giving blood, urinating in cups (can we please have larger cups, seriously?), having ultrasounds, participating in very awkward conversations about all my private body parts, and having doctors question me over and over and over again about my symptoms. They talk over me, at me, but never *to* me about what's going on with my body. In fact, scarily, they don't seem to know what's going on, and that worries me a lot. They're supposed to be the experts.

But here I am, back in hospital again, sitting in a pair of loose shorts and a baggy burgundy T-shirt that has the Ripcurl logo on it because, like most Aussie kids, I think surf brands are the peak of sophistication. Like all teens, I am very concerned with how I look. I have always been petite, but I am starting to look exceptionally gaunt now. Unprepared for this hospital visit, I have checked in with hairy legs, and I feel very self-conscious about this. Probably because this time, as I check into the hospital ward, I notice that I'm being watched like a hawk in a way that feels intrusive and judgmental. Every piece of food that goes down (and inevitably comes back up or out) is documented, and I am followed to and from the bathroom, down those long, sterile cream-colored hospital corridors with zero privacy. I pee and poop with the door slightly ajar and always with an adult nearby.

The "bed rest" I am told will be helpful for me seems elusive to obtain in the hospital. I am awakened every twenty minutes or so by a flashlight being shone into my eyes, so my blood pressure can be checked, and so that new bags of unidentifiable liquids can be attached to the tube and needle in my hand. Doctors and nurses come in and out in a steady stream and look at my body. They talk to each other about me, but they don't actually talk *to* me. It's as if I'm transparent or a ghost.

This isn't the first medical trip like this I've encountered, and over the last year, throughout visits to hospitals, specialists, and doctors' offices, I've heard so many variations of what supposedly could be wrong with me. Everything from "It's just a stomach bug," to "It could be an ulcer," to "It's reflux," or "It's just stress," as well as the old classic "There's nothing wrong with you; it's just in your head." The last one has been said more times than I can count.

When I check into the ward, I am given a blue sheet of paper with questions on it to answer for the medical staff. It comes with a chart that shows little faces in circles to indicate levels of happiness or unhappiness. I am asked to match what I am feeling to the corresponding face I associate it with. I am bluntly honest on the form. I am not in a good place. I am deeply upset and scared that this is the peak of my life and things are never going to get any better. I figure the more I tell them, the easier it should be for them to help me. All I want is an answer. I want to know what is wrong with me.

Once I have handed this form in, I am visited by a couple of doctors who ask more probing questions about what I eat and when, and question me vigorously when I mention I am in pain all over my body as though they are looking for a kind of "proof" I seem unable to provide. They look at each other as if they can't compute my answers. You see, I was expecting this honesty of mine to help them find the logical answer to what was happening to me, but as it turns out, it seems to have steered them the wrong way. They've taken my sadness and fear and my inability to eat properly due to my pain and nausea to mean something entirely different from what I know it to be. The fun new label being thrown around, among others, is "eating disorder," so when I'm being watched by the medical team, it's actually more like spying. They don't understand how much I have internalized my pain and sickness, how "normal" this abnormal situation has become for me. The more I have to defend myself, the warier I become of the medical staff. I feel betrayed by them, and I no longer trust them to help me. I don't even know if this potential new diagnosis of an eating disorder was mentioned to my parents, but for some reason, I now feel like I have done something wrong and don't mention it to them when they visit me. I don't feel like a human being anymore. I am now considered "sick." I am an annoying puzzle with pieces missing, a burden, a bother, a number, a patient, but definitely not human.

The assumption is I'm either doing something wrong or I am stressed. I don't ever recall feeling as though the medical professionals acknowledged that *I was suffering*, very scared, and in need of help. I offer up a range of suggestions of what my sickness could be, primarily because I don't feel I am being listened to, that I am not being taken seriously. But I am dismissed or questioned, and every insight I try to give about what is happening is overlooked. I am convinced that the medical professionals are missing the point—that *I* am the one living like this, and *I know my body better than they do*. I know what is happening is not normal and can't be explained away with a shrug. I know I'm not making any of my symptoms up, but I also know that when I describe it, the list is so long that it does sound like a farcical script.

I know that when I rattle off the entirety of what I am feeling physically at times, the adults get this glazed look over their faces, their mouths seem to tighten up, and I can see that it bothers or frustrates them. When I say that my whole body hurts; that anything I eat causes me pain, vomiting, or diarrhea; that my skin sometimes hurts; that my eyes smart; that my mouth is constantly filled with ulcers; that my neck is so tight it feels like my head will snap off if I turn it; that the word *tired* doesn't come close to the fatigue I feel; that my head pounds relentlessly; that there are so many types of pain going on in my gut that are new to me, ranging from sharp and stabbing to dull and cramping, that it feels like there is liquid fire in my throat and huge bulges that form in my stomach and move around and then disappear again; that I feel like I am starting to lose my memory or my mind, as I forget things all the time and feel totally out of control; and so many other symptoms . . . Well, you, too, might have a glazed look just by reading that list.

I am also sick with colds, sinus infections, and other viruses repetitively, and I seem to go from one illness to the next without a gap. My life seems like a cycle of visits to doctors' offices where I am handed yet another prescription for antibiotics or told condescendingly that it "is not that bad." However, all the standard tests they've run just don't seem to add up to anything that makes sense to them.

I have done what was suggested—to press the button on the remote attached to my bed if I need help—because my stomach is as hard as a rock, swollen to the point it hurts to breathe, and the pain and nausea are intolerable. I am in relentless agony, and each time I let them know something is wrong, I am told I am constipated, or too stressed, or too young to be having these symptoms. Furthermore, I am told that I should be drinking more water and trying harder not to let myself become upset. All of the other pains I report seem to be ignored as irrelevant. It seems that, no matter what symptoms I face, they are my fault or I am too young to be experiencing them, and apparently, I should know this already.

I am aware that I am a difficult puzzle that the doctors need to solve, and as my symptoms can vary from minute to minute, I know they think I am making it hard for them to do their job. In fact, this has been expressed to me many times in varying forms. "Oh, you are a tricky one, aren't you?" "You are not making our job easy," and "If you would just eat something, you would probably feel better and we might not be trying to work this out for you, young lady," often delivered with a wry smile, are the kinds of comments physicians and nurses make when I vocalize anything I am feeling. As a result, I feel like I need to apologize for being so complicated, even though *I* am the one actually living this experience. I desperately wish for the doctors to have to live this way for a day, to have some idea of what this feels like. I think if they did, they'd be doing a lot more to help me.

Stress, which the doctors sometimes refer to as being a cause of my issues—and which is definitely ever-present at this time—is the result of this agonizing, sickening feeling that is all over my body constantly and not knowing what it is. I truly believe that my stress is not the cause, it's just a symptom. But getting the adults around me to actually listen to me, and take action when I explain this seems to be a total no-go. I didn't feel stressed until I became a "sick" person. It happened in that order, not the other way around.

A gamut of tests has been run over the past year, but out of all the tests and procedures, the day that sticks out the most in my mind's eye is the day of my barium meal procedure, a routine procedure used to diagnose a variety of different things inside the digestive tract. It involved my drinking a large quantity of exceptionally cold, thick liquid barium, a type of metal, through a straw while lying flat on my back in a brightly lit room. Forcing the barium down was really difficult for me. If you've ever had a hangover and then tried to gulp down a thick shake while lying down in the summer sun, you will know how I felt at that moment. If you haven't, I wouldn't advise trying it! Although I am unsure of how, I did it and patiently waited for the test to begin.

To me, the idea seemed to be that a group of technicians would observe the barium as it moved through my gut via a monitor in a room close by, helping them to spot potential causes of my symptoms. The four adults in the room talked among themselves about the day-to-day things they were doing, giggling, never looking me in the eye or explaining why they were occupying my space. They were at work, doing what coworkers do.

I felt really lonely and scared, but I had been warned that I wasn't allowed to move, so I just lay as still as I could. The longer I was there, the more the nausea and the pain in my gut seemed to worsen. And the worse the pain in my gut got, the more the rest of my body started to scream. My head was pounding. I could feel sweat running down my neck. I felt like an elephant was sitting on my bladder. Pain radiated through my lower back, my neck, my shoulders, and my inner thighs. I felt like I was going to be sick. I called out that I didn't feel good and I wanted someone to assist me. Without the technicians ever looking my way, one of them used the microphone in the booth to speak to me in the treatment room.

"Your gut is just being *waaay* too slow. You can't throw up, or we will have to start again. Just lie still."

I didn't know I could have a *slow* gut, but the tone of her voice suggested that if I did, it would absolutely be my fault, and I definitely was not allowed to throw up because it would be a major inconvenience for her. I blinked back tears and breathed through the waves of nausea. As I concentrated on not being sick, the technicians left the booth and entered the room. In one of the men's hands was what I can only describe now as a length of wood with a padded piece of blue foam taped to one end. He told me that the barium wasn't moving through my guts very well, so he had to help it along by putting pressure on my stomach and intestines with the padded plank.

He used the spongy end of the plank to push down and drag the barium through my gut, trying to force the barium to move through my digestive system. I genuinely believe he was trying to be gentle, but I was in so much pain that I whimpered as he pushed on my abdomen. As soon as I made a noise, one of the other men said, "Come on now. Be brave," in a slightly upbeat tone as though maybe he was trying to get me to laugh at the situation. But I was too scared and in too much pain to take it as a joke, and frankly, I thought I was already being very brave, and now I thought I was weak. It was an intense experience, not being able to move, with adults I had never met hovering over me, pressing down on me, and not being allowed to make a noise. I felt truly helpless. Once the technicians seemed satisfied with their prodding and poking, they walked back into their booth and continued talking about their day, paying me no mind.

After some time of lying still and trying not to move, I was advised that the test was over, and I was taken by an orderly back to my hospital bed. I was exhausted and nauseated. I quickly turned my light out and got under the covers, hoping to get some sleep without throwing up all the barium in my gut. I hadn't been in my bed for more than half an hour when I heard the hospital staff gather outside my closed bed curtain.

Man: "According to the notes, she's been complaining of a lot of pain and isn't eating, and her bowel movements have no pattern. She

10

has barely eaten anything since she was checked into the ward. She's been in the ER before, and they suggested it was stress and then sent her home. Possibly an eating disorder given her age and continuing weight loss. I mean, you can see she's really, really skinny."

Female: "She's a teenage girl. I've seen it all before."

They made knowing, smug noises of agreement.

I was lying on my side as they opened the curtain, trying so hard not to cry, but despite my best efforts, a couple of tears rolled down my face, which they did not acknowledge. My hands were clenched. I felt humiliated, enraged, and weak. The voice in my head was screaming, "Help me! I just need you to help me. I don't need you to judge me, just HELP ME!" But I said nothing because I knew it wouldn't help. It had been made clear that my voice didn't count. For the next few minutes, I tried to focus on looking brave. They gave me a basic run-of-the-mill check-in, which essentially told me they didn't know anything much yet and that I would be spending the coming days pooping out solid white heavy barium that might not flush easily. Oh, the joy.

I nodded in acknowledgment because, at that moment, I actually couldn't speak. I felt like I couldn't use my mouth at all. Words failed me for the first time in my life. I was angry. I was terrified. Frankly, I was fed up, but mainly I was crushed because I just wanted to know what was going on and I was sick of being sick. They asked if I wanted the light turned back on, and I shook my head no. After they closed the curtain, I curled up in a ball and cried deeply, and I silently screamed into my pillow as though I was grieving because I was. I was grieving who I had been before that moment. I knew I had been changed and that I wasn't ever going back to being the person I had been before. Whatever I had been, whatever path I had been on up to that point, fractured. Like some cosmic shift or a movement underneath me like the plates of the earth changing position, I, too, changed in an irreversible way.

I felt invisible for the first time in my life. It changed who I was and who I could have become. I had learned that I was insignificant, that my experience wasn't real enough. My pain wasn't real enough, or justified enough, and if people couldn't see what was happening to me, then they couldn't see **me** at all.

WELLNESS TIP:
Alpha-cise

Ever get that triggered, panicky feeling where your mind is racing and you can feel your entire body tingle as it takes on whatever you're unable to stop thinking about?

When the mind runs away and sets off physical symptoms, it's time to give the mind something to focus on. That nervous energy needs to be directed somewhere! Taking the alphabet from *A* to *Z* and a category like Foods, run through your alphabet, finding a food that starts with each letter. You can change the category as many times as you like and run through the alphabet from start to finish until the sense of panic has left your body and your mind settles down a notch.

It might go something like this:

A for *Apple*,

B for *Banana*,

C for *Carrot*,

D for *Dragon fruit* . . .

and so on till *Z*. Then start from the top with a new category till you find your equilibrium again.

2

THE POWER OF WORDS

Crohn's disease and *irritable bowel syndrome:* a punishing disease that compromises the immune system and a fickle syndrome, both affecting the digestive system in different ways. Both misunderstood. Both awful. Both now my burdens. These terms meant nothing to me when I first heard them. They bounced around my brain like empty, hollow globes of air. The only thing I really heard when I was finally diagnosed with these incurable conditions was "I am not crazy." I sat in the doctors' office in a daze. I didn't feel relieved. No, I felt vindicated and angry. I clenched my hands as tightly as I could in an effort not to scream. I **knew that I should never have been made to feel the way I did.** I knew my body, and I had fought for her when no one was listening. The hurt was unimaginable. My soul burned with torment.

I'd lived under all three labels; undiagnosed, diagnosed and misdiagnosed, and each journey had come at a price. I had been left altered, angry, grief-stricken and baffled that those sworn to do no harm had blamed me for my illness and ignored my words, which likely would have led to me being accurately diagnosed in the first place. I was sent out of the hospital thinking I had an overly acidic stomach and a slow gut whose onset was caused by stress. I knew that was wrong. It translated to my having to take handfuls of tablets that, sadly, made me more unwell because I was treating an issue I did not have. Left with no other choice, I was chewing down strong pain medication daily like it was candy, just to get a couple of bearable hours out of the day, not knowing that this was contributing to the constipation and pain. I eventually discovered that I had irritable bowel syndrome and was then being pumped full of laxatives and other things that only hindered my healing because they only treated part of the problem and, as was later discovered, were inflaming my gut instead of healing it. I pushed forward, at times feeling like I was walking over broken glass in the process, until I heard the word *Crohn's*. It took far too long for the doctors to reconcile that I had both Crohn's Disease and Irritable Bowel Syndrome at the same time despite me raising the idea countless times; a frustrating and trying journey in and of itself.

I'd like to tell you that things were simpler from there, but they weren't. The medications I was prescribed proved to be as pain- and stress-inducing as the disease itself, and I came close to being dependent on steroids, painkillers, sleeping pills, and antidepressants to function, but it was not functional at all; it was absolutely agonizing and not a way I could live. The side effects of every pill and injection made me feel as though I was now being punished for seeking treatment. There was no relief. If anything, my path became filled with even more obstacles. I eventually learned, through a lot of painful trial and error, that my body hates pharmaceuticals, especially steroids and almost all painkillers. Truly *hates* them! And the extremity of my gut issues means I often can't even break them down and absorb them in the first place! The damage I was doing to my organs by swallowing them was taking a toll on me in every imaginable way.

Long before getting to a complete and accurate diagnosis I was put in touch with a Naturopath for symptom management as what had been offered to me medically seemed to make me more unwell. As a result, I leaned towards natural therapies even though I was told that it was ridiculous to do so. My body simply responds better to them, though I use pharmaceuticals as and if needed alongside naturopathy to keep control of the situation. I believe each of us has different needs, and it's worth being open to both methods so you can assess what helps you. What I know is that naturopathy is an approach that works for me—a real night-and-day difference compared to pharmaceutical methods alone.

It was a truly exhausting roller-coaster ride to be on, and by the time the and best therapies for me were found, the damage had already been done. I was obviously sick physically, but I was also profoundly unwell mentally and emotionally.

In large part, at that time, I was sent off into the world with absolutely no idea of what my body was doing or how to live with it. The feeling of invisibility really set in, and life was tough. *Invisible* isn't just a term or a feeling. It's a label that becomes a state of mind, one which began to erode me from the inside out. It undermined every positive thought I had ever had about myself, my body, and my life, and all the possibilities I had imagined for myself seemed to fall away.

There is only so long a person can withstand the process of looking for a diagnosis. There are only so many times a person can be told to consume things that cause them irreparable pain. There is only so much that a person can withstand when they are hurt, scared, and find themselves with no voice. **Getting a full, or even partial diagnosis, does not magically erase what led up to it.** I had swallowed trauma after trauma, unable to understand it or process it. The pressure inside me developed day by day until my body could no longer contain it. The wave I had been riding for so long finally crashed, and what was left behind as the whitewash pulled away from the shore was a shell of a person. I was both entirely numb and full of anguish. That's when my mind and emotions took control of me in ways I never knew were possible.

I found myself developing strange habits and having thoughts that wouldn't go away. I started to count everything, from the number of times I chewed food to the number of times I brushed my hair. I washed my hands over and over until my skin cracked open and bled. I carried antibacterial soap in a container with me, even when I went to school (long before hand sanitizer was a normal thing—I was such a trendsetter!). I'd go into a complete state of meltdown if something in my bedroom was moved from where I had placed it, even though my room was so messy it often looked like a bomb had hit it. I was so terrified of becoming sick because I feared sickness might actually kill me now. I didn't yet understand that my condition had an effect on my immune system, that in fact my condition was considered an autoimmune disease, but I had noticed that I seemed to get ill more often and that the common cold no longer felt like just a cold. Sickness now hit me with an intensity no one around me seemed to be able to recognise or relate to. When I was ill, my entire body would be screaming at me in pain, from my skin and muscles to my stomach, and when I *was* what many of us with chronic illness call "normie" sick (sick with an illness everyone gets), it was almost impossible for me to remember simple details or put words together in the right order as my brain turned to mush, let alone control my emotions. I didn't yet understand the cognitive effects of my condition either.

In my mind, it had become a chain of cause and effect, and I was convinced that if I did not wash my hands four times or if the stuffed toy sitting on my shelf wasn't on a perfect ninety-degree angle, I would be inviting something terrible to happen to me. I had come out of hospital entirely believing that I had caused this to happen to me, that I had done something bad and was being punished for it. I felt like I was being hunted down by something. As you may be suspecting, I had developed obsessive-compulsive disorder.

I believe it was a way for my mind to try to cope and gain some kind of control over what was going on inside, and sometimes I just didn't know how to vocalize my experience in a way that anyone else could understand. I was extremely anxious, I had panic attacks, and I quickly spiraled into a desperate state of depression. I was having what I now know were PTSD episodes, like flashbacks, from the trauma of repeated misdiagnosis, having my body pushed and pulled over and over again, and basically being treated like I was somehow making this happen to myself. I couldn't sleep, partly from pain and partly from fear. My body and my mind became dark and scary places to reside. I didn't trust my body anymore, and I couldn't trust my mind. I am positive most of this presented as some kind of teenage angst.

My family, whom I treasure, did all they could to help me by taking me to doctors and surgeons, counselors and psychiatrists, and naturopaths (when it was still taboo to see a holistic health professional, and I am thankful every day that they did). Without them, I would have made a devastating and permanent choice. I am here in no small part because their desire to find solutions never wavered. They gave me a gift that I will never be able to fully repay.

They presented a brave face through all of this process, but I could see in their eyes the stress that it placed them under. I wanted so badly to be well so I could stop the stress they were going through. I didn't want my parents visiting me in the hospital or having me cry on their shoulders to be the way they saw their child. I wanted them to see me—the full me that included so much more than my symptoms.

I will never forget a moment I had in the car with my dad during this time. I was crying, as I felt so sick and so sad, and my dad held me tightly and said, "I would walk through fire if it meant I could make this better. I am here." It broke my heart, but made me love him even more. My hero.

What a blessing it was that I had them all there at my side. I know so many people with invisible illnesses who never had that. I am one of the lucky ones. They made sure I had someone to talk to and were willing to look outside the box and into alternative medicine as well as the westernized style. Mum and Dad and Sis, thank you for all that you did. You saved my life.

Thankfully, I was being treated by a counselor, but my experience was so layered because of all the ongoing diagnosis, misdiagnosis and no-diagnosis phases, that progressing mentally and emotionally was slow. In fact, I was so regressed that the counselor would have me draw pictures and use a sandpit with toys to create images of what I was feeling. This is a technique often used with small children when they can't verbalize what they have experienced. I was a teenager going to high school, but I was using Barbie dolls in a sandpit in a counselor's office to try to help me process what I was experiencing, grieve what I had lost, and understand the list of mental illnesses I was rapidly accumulating. That's how bad things had become for me.

I didn't know how to explain to teachers and friends why I had to run from class to the bathroom, or, worse, to vomit just outside one because I couldn't get to the toilet in time—yes, this has happened—or that I was unable to follow along with some of the lessons because it was like my brain just wouldn't work anymore. The times I tried to explain to people at school or in my classes what was going on in my life, I was shot down with comments like "Whatever. You look fine," or "Shut up. I would kill to be as skinny as you," or "Get over it already. You aren't dying," or "I don't want to hear about this. It's gross." I quickly refrained from talking to people. I spent a lot of time outside of class crying. I was bullied endlessly for being so skinny, for being so emotional, and for my behavior that often followed a pain or symptom flare. I was on an emotional roller coaster that I couldn't get off, and I was trying to manage physical symptoms that I didn't understand with a mind I was unable to control.

Please cue your mental image of a barely five-foot-tall, skinny girl with dyed-red hair, wearing dog collars to school paired with heavy black eyeliner, a pair of high-top Converse, shapeless clothes, and a sulky look on her face—that was me in a nutshell. In fact, at that point in my life, if somebody asked me how I was, I would actually respond with "I'm still alive, so you tell me." Yeah, I was heaps of fun to be around!

I had been labeled "invisible" by the world, and everything I observed seemed to reinforce that this was the box I had been put in for life. The only reference to my illnesses within the world around me seemed to be on TV and in film, where characters like me were stereotyped as "nuts", and their symptoms were made out to be some kind of annoying or amusing personal choice. They were always blamed for their condition, and were shown as not deserving of care. I suddenly found the world telling me that because I was sick and had mental illnesses I was weak, pathetic, and "wrong". I was some kind of embarrassment. I was something to be ashamed of; something to hide; something to laugh at. I know that when ones condition often involves pooping, gas, bleeding, massive bloating, vomiting, burping and making mistakes when speaking, it doesn't make for the smoothest conversation starter! But why not? It's all so much more common than you might think! Most people don't exactly sit down over a meal and casually talk about the mucous falling out of their butthole and into their pants.

To make matters worse, these issues can't be seen with the naked eye. So when you keep telling others that you're in pain, agony, and feel too sick to go out or even talk, people eventually start to question your sanity and loyalty, and you soon find that your friendship circles shrink dramatically. I found myself met with terms like *weak, pathetic*, and *too sensitive*. I was told over and over again to "toughen up" or to "grow a thicker skin and get over it already." These things were often said by people who wanted to protect me. However, they didn't realize that what they were saying was reinforcing this invisibility box that I now found myself living in.

While I griped, grumbled, and sometimes was just a big depressing mess of emotions, I just couldn't find a way to talk about this enough to find sustainable coping strategies because the world around me didn't want to hear about it. My strategy at the time was to bury it in a box, as deep down in my mind as I possibly could. Of course, this actually made me acutely unwell, but I didn't understand that at the time.

One of the biggest dilemmas was that I didn't have a single example of anyone even close to my age who was living with any of my invisible illnesses to look to for hope, guidance, or support. No one around me knew what my conditions were. I had never heard of any kind of foundation or support group for these diseases whatsoever, though I am proudly an ambassador for one now. Those living examples I needed may very well have been out there, but their own invisibility and stigma meant that they went unnoticed by me.

I can't place enough emphasis on the damage all of this did to me and how many years I then worked, and still do, to change my own opinion of myself and my place in the world.

Now, I know this may feel like a big overshare on my part, telling you all this, but it is for an important reason. It is because of what I was learning, and it was a lesson I didn't expect to get. Yes, I had learned that being invisible was hard and that I was clearly not going to get a simple run at life. I was never going to be "normal" and might never be accepted as I was. That was abundantly clear, and it was scary, but I didn't know that I was also getting a crash course in representation. I didn't realize that life was handing me a whopper of a lesson, one which so many of us need to learn: it is essential know that we are safe, seen, valued and heard. To know that who we are and what we are is accepted. We all need connection to someone or something, that directly relates to who we know ourselves to be on the inside. I didn't know that I was learning the power of the word *invisible*, or the power of words in general, for that matter (which may seem surprising because those that know me . . . well, they know I am all about words and I can talk the legs off of a chair).

I am aware now that words count, they matter. When each of us opens our mouth and speaks, we have the power to change the course of someone's life. For better or worse. How we are labeled matters. How we label *ourselves* really matters throughout life. In adulthood, we choose labels for ourselves. We empower ourselves with them. We sometimes wear them as a costume. We will even just try them on for size. We inevitably build our lives, careers, and businesses around them. We adjust our health, both physical and mental, when we are triggered to do so by specific labels and terms. Your very identity is an accumulation of labels chosen by you and given to you by others, which develops into journeys and life experiences that have either reinforced or broken them for you. If I'd been able to see someone like me, with the same label, going out and carrying on in their pursuit of living a happy life, I would likely be a completely different person than who I am today.

So many painful years of self-discovery might have been replaced by special moments that created joyous memories instead. There are huge chunks of my life missing in my memory because they were so painful my mind hid them from me. If I had known it was OK to be who I was, maybe that would not have happened. If you think back over your own life right now can you identify the words, the labels, and the representations that have molded you? It's kind of amazing in reflection how we get to be the people that we are, isn't it? Quite often we don't even question the person we have become. It can feel like life just happened to us.

When words were crushing me, I turned to my imagination and creative outlets to cope. I read a copious amount of books and listened to more music than I can ever quantify. I did acting lessons, dance lessons, and music lessons. These lessons allowed me to play with words, to speak things I couldn't say in my real voice, to let it out through my body, to mold myself into another version of who I really was. I was no longer *me*, I was a gangster or a pilot or a funny character. Every role allowed me to build myself as a different person, one that was free of the pain and sickness and panic. And through these pathways, I was being applauded by audiences instead of pitied or judged for who I was in my real life. I gripped on to this for dear life, not knowing I was learning to survive by being a chameleon of sorts. I didn't know at the time that this harsh lesson would turn into one of the greatest gifts I would ever get.

Today, when I think about it all, my ability to adapt, to transform, feels like a superpower because I can choose to drop one label and pick up another one with relative ease. I'm not bound to my career titles and descriptions in the same way as most people that I meet, because I never assume anyone sees *me* in the first place. I know now that the lessons I've learned have allowed me to wear so many labels: professional dancer, choreographer, receptionist, project manager, stage director, producer, founder, CEO, wife, bisexual, ambassador, victim, leader, follower, wellness coach, and more. I am all of them and none of them. I transform when I want to and when I need to. However, I am not fake. It is not an act when I transform. It is simply me bringing out another piece of my authentic self. I am not attached to any singular bit of me. It is all real and relevant, but I am in control of how I use it.

Yes, words are powerful. I see both sides of this coin. Words can break or mold you in so many ways. The choice is yours. But here's the rub: for many people, making that choice is overwhelming, too overwhelming, actually, because the words they hear and the labels they are given may land on them *before* they've had an opportunity to build their resilience and have it fortified by self-analysis and experience. Frankly, if they have no example, no representation, to turn to in their darkest moments, those words and labels can crush them. Some of these people will make it through and fortify their resilience through self-analysis and their own investigation into their humanness, but some may not make it through this at all, which is a tragedy that could be prevented.

While I am grateful for the lessons I've learned from my invisibility, I don't want anyone else to have to experience it. My heart shatters when I know someone is at the starting line of that lifelong race against the world. Without my experience with it, I doubt I would have thrown caution to the wind to live this crazy life of mine. So I am proud to don the cape of invisibility because I know I can't be defined by any one word. I have changed my attachment to it by dedicating much of my life to understanding who I am and what I am capable of with and without the labels the world places on me. The world may think I'm invisible, but *I see me*, and that's what counts.

When the world labels us and we bury ourselves in our acceptance of it, we suffer. We all have differences. **Those differences are not there to suffocate us, they are there to elevate us.** Embracing our differences is what allows us to roll with the waves of life instead of being battered by them. Differences are what allow us to keep learning, keep evolving, and keep up with life instead of preventing ourselves from experiencing it. How silly of us to believe it is worth wasting this precious life on fitting our being under one neat little label or title just because it was handed to us, rather than encouraging each other to experiment and use the skills and differences that are innate to us to succeed and live well. How cruel to teach people that sickness of any kind makes them less valuable or less loveable than anyone else!

Will *invisible* be with me for life? Yes, it probably will. Society has decided to place me there, but that doesn't mean it is my only label, and it doesn't mean that I have to take that label as a drastic life sentence, which is definitely where I started out. I can see this label as an opportunity to live with one foot in the grave and accept the shame the world wants me to carry, or I can define my own future for myself. I can take the word and redefine it just enough to let me be freer than many of the people I know who don't have much to rebel against in the first place. That is what I choose to do every day of the week.

Whether you like it or not, you are living in some kind of box under some type of label. Society reinforces your labels and will, for the most part, encourage you to stay safely, exactly where you are. Some of you are convinced that it's too risky to try on another one for size, that it's too hard, or that you are not worthy of another. So if you are waiting for permission, grant it for yourself right now. Work out who the hell you are!

What makes you shine? We all have something. If you can't shake the label you already have, then ask yourself what it has taught you and how you can use that lesson to make your life, or someone else's, better. That's the question I asked myself. Work out how to use your thing, whatever it is, instead of covering it up. Let yourself change. You're going to anyway! You will have experiences that will change you constantly. You will learn new things year after year, whether it's from a hospital bed, a boardroom, or your interactions with others. Please don't define yourself by one word, burying the best of yourself in the process. Don't let yourself be squashed by the need to conform to one word. Be all the words, or none of them, or a variety of them. Live. Your. Life. Unapologetically live it as only *you* can.

What I have taken away from a couple of decades of battle with myself, with labels, and with the world are a few things that I think are worth summarizing. Not one person you know is actually defined by one label alone. Their job, their role, their label isn't all there is. They are a multitude of things, as are you. Try to remember that the next time someone speaks to you or enters your life, especially if you don't share their life experience. The invisible folks like me, for example, are not invisible at all, so help them feel visible. Every single person on the planet has a desire to be recognised by someone else for exactly who they are, in their fully rounded, entirely whole humanness. Start conversations, ask questions, and get curious about others and other ways of living. If you don't have one yourself, you likely know many people who have an invisible disease or a chronic pain condition, and just aren't aware of it because they feel like they will be shamed or treated as "less than" if they tell you. The more we categorize people under one label and refuse to delve deeper, the longer we force whole sections of society to suffer silently. If you have the privilege—and it is a privilege—of being one of the socially acceptable, visible people, don't enable each other to keep the rest of us invisible. We need your help to change that over time. If the disease I have described, or any other, sounds gross to you, perhaps imagine having to live with it before you pass judgment. Let's all approach each other with a little perspective.

My fellow invisible buddies could offer the world so much if only society made room for them too. It starts with you being willing to check in with the people you know and ask, "Have you ever heard of invisible disease?" You can help normalize instead of stigmatize. We need you. But you need us too, probably more than you know. We are resilient and strong in a deeper way because we face adversity every day. You need people like that in your life, your business, your school, and your friendship circles. You need people like that making some of the big decisions in the world because we truly understand how challenging life can be and the difference between surviving and living. You can learn a lot from us that would make you better at everything you do and every relationship you have. Disease doesn't equal *defective* or *less than*. A battle with disease shows strength. So let's bust some labels and transform! In doing so, we are more inclined to have empathy and kindness at the forefront of how we deal with people instead of fear or indifference, and that can only mean a nicer world for all of us to live in. Idealistic? Yes. Worth doing your bit? Absolutely!

Regardless of what you face in life, it is my most sincere hope that over time as your own life develops, it takes you whole paragraphs, maybe even pages, to summarize who you are instead of just one or two labels that society has picked for you. Please remember that you are complex, varied, learning, growing, changing, adapting, and rallying all the time. You are human, and only you get to define *your* labels.

When someone bravely tells you that they are experiencing something you do not personally understand, when they tell you of their pain, illness, trauma, or differences, please, for the love of all that is good in the world, respond with care. Your opinion of someone else's lived experience truly doesn't count, and it is not your right to project your feelings onto them to preserve your own imagined view of the world. When someone explains their lived experience, the first response, whether it's from a doctor, friend, or colleague, should be to believe the person and to lead with empathy, not to interrogate and judge them. People are capable of empathy, even if they disagree with each other. No matter what you think of someone or their situation, please, please start there. And the next time you go to label someone else or treat them differently because of a word, remember that they have a right to their own self-descriptive paragraphs and pages of words, just like you do, and that you do not get to define those for someone else. Ever.

WELLNESS TIP:
Check on Your Body

Please take a moment to honor your body, as it's not just your brain facilitating your reading right now.

If you can, roll your shoulders back six times in a row to feel the muscles relax and soften.

Gently take your right arm and lift it above your head, bend the arm at the elbow, and place your right hand just above your left ear. Breathe in deeply through your nose, and as you exhale out of your mouth, gently stretch your neck by bringing your right ear towards your right shoulder. Hold this position for at least ten seconds, breathing deeply and continually.

Repeat this for the left side of your neck too, changing arms accordingly.

Repeat this from the top three times.

Now that you have increased blood flow to your muscles and given your body a good dose of oxygen, empowering it to work while increasing your sense of calm, you are ready for the next lesson.

3

SELF-CARE IS ESSENTIAL

Around the world, there has historically been this style of thinking that states that taking care of oneself is weak or silly or selfish. While I will happily scream from the rooftops now that this thinking is ridiculous, unrealistic, and damaging to the world, I probably fell into that camp of thinking myself for a short period of my life. Bottling things up and acting fine and having a big blowout over the weekend was more my style for a while. I just didn't know anything else. Nowadays, though, self-care, the notion of actually looking after oneself, has been gaining popularity, but it is often confused with self-indulgence. And that's certainly how my experience with self-care and wellness started.

Coming out of my complex younger years, I chose to continue pursuing one of my passions—dance—and that meant I was placing extraordinary pressure on my body and using both my emotional and mental health to create dynamic performances. While there were enormous benefits in that for me, I was also placing my future, my income, and my resources on top of a body that needed specialized care to be able to function. I calculated that obvious risk and pursued it with my teeth out, but the process of sharing so much of me left my tank personally empty. Having to fake my way through days of agony and illness just so I could show up and teach a class or get to perform was becoming exhausting. It was becoming an issue that I could no longer ignore.

Being sick at work was affecting my ability to keep the lights on and a roof over my head. I needed to look after my body differently because what I was doing, which was quite a lot like any other dance professional, wasn't cutting it any longer. Coming out of those early years, I had dissociated from my body. I felt betrayed by it, so I had got to the point that I saw it as an entirely separate entity to myself. It didn't feel like *me*, and I definitely didn't like the way it looked. I was constantly comparing my body to everyone else's, wishing for it to be different than what it was. Dissociating is a type of self-protection that can happen when you have experienced trauma. I severed the ties to my body emotionally, which made it feel easier on the surface to deal with my body when it threw a curveball at me, like extreme fatigue or inflamed joints. However, the reality is that self-protection turned into an ugly curse because the situation I experienced wasn't temporary. Being sick and in pain and stressed about it was not going to magically stop for me. So that dissociation was creating issues by its very nature.

Through dance, I had been learning and developing an intense connection to my physical form in the sense of how it worked mechanically, and I had a vested interest in protecting it for the sake of my career. I started to look for ways to do just that.

My first point of call was all about physical maintenance. I created this extreme "hour of power" for myself daily, which included running five to eight kilometers, doing a few hundred crunches, and working on my flexibility so I could do the splits, high kicks, and aerial maneuvers. This was on top of the four to eight hours of dancing I was already doing by teaching, rehearsing, choreographing, and performing. My hour of power was driven by my need to say to my body, "Hey, listen up, I have control, and if I want you to do one hundred crunches, you're going to do it," which was the obsessive part of my brain at work, and because I had a real chip on my shoulder about being less physically capable than my counterparts. Dancers around me were doing similar things, and they seemed strong, so I wanted to do the same. The hour of power was over the top, but I also knew these exercises would keep my balance strong, protect parts of my spine and hips, and maintain my endurance and stamina. These things are practically an insurance policy for any dancer, but anxiety and stress still played a significant role in my life, as did PTSD, and my hour of power sometimes increased the barrage of negativity in my head and the pain in my body. It seemed to have the opposite effect on me than it did on other people.

I didn't always create movements that suited me or conveyed what I wanted to express. So sometimes there wasn't an outlet for what *I* was feeling. My ability to feed myself as a dancer (no small feat, even though I have small feet—sorry, I couldn't help myself!) was now also connected to what a director, dance studio owners, and an audience were willing to pay to see.

Not feeling like you have an outlet or a way to recharge may seem familiar to you, like it did to me. By the time you have done your work and talked to your team, fed your kids and your spouse, done the housework, and checked in on your friends, (or if you are chronically ill you might have battled to get one of those things done), then your tank might be sitting on empty, and yet you just keep on going, practically running on fumes. Most people live like this. You know that you only have a few more liters of fuel in the tank, but you never head to the service station to refill. Like many of you, I've been trained by society to satisfy others or my responsibilities long before I satisfy myself. And back then, when I refilled the tank, I picked the cheapest petrol and the smallest amount possible. In fact, I wouldn't even turn the damned engine off to refuel! I would practically roll in, hang my body out of the car window so I could reach the petrol hose, attach it to the side of the car for a split second, and be on the road before noticing if I had got all the fuel I needed, which I never did!

In that vein, the next thing I did when I recognized I needed something to refuel me was to select the cheapest thing I could think of. I purchased nail polish, some out-of-the-bottle black hair dye, and the lowest-cost beauty mask I could find; gave myself half an hour or so to apply them; camped out in front of the television; and convinced myself that this would be enough. For an hour or so I felt pretty good about myself (and I discovered how good I looked with black hair, a look I kept for way too long), but later that night, I felt the same as I had before. I went back to living on fumes, unimpressed by my experiment. But a few weeks later, I decided to get a massage. Having little idea what to look for in a therapist, I went to one of those generic massage places you find in a shopping center. The massage was enjoyable, but it really didn't scratch the surface of what my body needed. My muscles and joints were naturally very inflamed, not just from dancing but from the inflammation in my body brought on by Crohn's disease. Again, I felt pretty good after the massage, but the following day, I felt the same as before, and so I went back to that fume existence.

The following month, I went shopping in a secondhand clothing store for some updated looks. I didn't have the money to buy new clothes; I was a paycheck-to-paycheck queen. I hoped that getting a fresh look might perk me up and help me feel fulfilled. And it did . . . for about an hour. I may have looked like the ultimate hipster-chic, slightly Goth, not-afraid-to-rock-a-lapel-and-some-sequins girl, but it didn't move the needle. I noticed that I got a big rush of happiness as I left with a bag full of items. But the following day I was back to square one, if not square zero.

In reflection, I now know that this was self-indulgence. I wasn't doing anything consistently. I wasn't doing anything I could **sustain** regularly. My body had no way of normalizing any of this hit-and-miss behavior. What I was doing was getting a dopamine rush of chemical awesome in the brain that made my body feel satisfied short-term because it was activating the reward center of my brain. But as we all know, what goes up must come down, and shortly after my initial rush, that's where I found myself—down. And down when you are already tired and sick is a low, low place to be. This became a critical lesson for me, and one I hope you will also embrace. Instant gratification, or self-indulgence (dopamine), is not how we are designed to function *all* the time. Do we need a bit of self-indulgence here and there? Yes. Do we need it a hundred times a day, like what we get from social media, stimulants, or pretty much anything that has a reward element to it? No. Dopamine does not magically refill itself instantaneously; it takes time and rest to do so, and continuous dopamine depletion can wreak havoc on the human form. Living like that is unsustainable for the body, and therefore the mind. Simple as that.

What I had gleaned from my short run of self-indulgent activity was that there was a direct chemical reaction to the activities I chose to do, and that reaction had a physical and emotional impact on my body and my perception of my life in that very moment. It sparked curiosity in me to research if there was a way to feel better for a longer term.

I found a massage clinic that specialized in working with athletes. Their treatment was undoubtedly more expensive, but being a dancer, I decided that I needed that kind of help. (Dancers *are hardcore athletes*.) Therefore, it made more sense to visit someone who specialized in what I did than to visit someone offering help to the general public.

Instead of being asked the surface-level questions like "Is this pressure OK?" I was asked, "What side of your body is most dominant? Are you more flexible on your left side? Are you moving dynamically or statically when you warm up? What anti-inflammatory foods are you consuming after a night of teaching dance? What are you doing to reduce lactic acid in your muscles?"

As the therapist worked on my body in a more strategic way, using my answers to their questions to guide the treatment, I found that I was unraveling some of the health secrets that my body was holding on to. As my body was treated, my mind was being educated. I started to draw connections between the questions I was asked and the reality I was living. I began to see that the specific type of movement I did or the kind of food I ate might play a deeper role in my well-being than I had understood up to that point—much deeper than just "do some exercise and eat a vegetable." I was getting down into the weeds and way outside my comfort zone, where all the good stuff in life actually comes from. I was starting to reconnect to my body emotionally, and I wasn't so much scared as I was curious about the impact that could have on me.

Going to generic fitness centers and seeing normal health professionals always seemed to lead to me having to explain (read: defend) my health situation. And that is, if I could make it to one! Half the time, I was too tired or sick to do these seemingly normal things. No one really understood how to work with someone like me. So I cast a much wider net to look for a group of holistic health specialists, like naturopaths, osteopaths, massage therapists, and so on, that could offer ways to treat me that were inclusive of everything that made up me and my life. And I needed to find things I could do from the comfort of my home, things I could do when I couldn't even get from the bedroom to the front door. I found in these professionals what I had never found in the traditional medical pros: a safe space where I could actually ask for help and know that I would receive it. Their energy and enthusiasm were infectious, and I started to open that door between my emotions and body even more! Naturopaths, in particular, were life-altering for me. They listened to every symptom, asked deep questions I had never been asked before, were attentive in a genuine and caring way, and were happy to work alongside any other professional, including traditional doctors. They never judged me, they just wanted to help me. They gave me light at the end of the tunnel, which finally wasn't a train.

Each session with them taught me more and more about my body, and they helped me edge forward with my mental and emotional health too. Slowly but surely, I started to recognize that my mental and emotional state could either help me cope better or it could hinder me dramatically, as a person, but even more so as someone with Crohn's. Finally, it dawned on me that the interconnected nature between my mind, body, and emotions was determining my quality of life. I couldn't leave out any part if I wanted to thrive. Ding, ding, ding! It was like a bell rang in my mind. I was as excited about it as Oprah is about giving out presents to an audience!

As this journey progressed and I sought out patterns and answers, it helped me feel more positive even when I faced setbacks. By paying close attention to how I felt, I discovered that the running I had added to my health routine as part of my hour of power was actually hindering me. Running is a great emotional-stress reliever and cardio exercise for many people, but it is also a higher inflammation-causing exercise, meaning my body wasn't able to cope with the added pressure, or the amount of cortisol it released in the process. I was already inflamed from my disease. I didn't need to add more inflammation on top of that. Where this would have previously deflated me, and I would have thrown in the towel altogether, I was able to see this insight as a huge win. Suddenly the negative things were positives. I felt elated. I was finally getting some answers! And those answers allowed me to make small tweaks to my lifestyle that helped me have a better quality of life.

Each exciting discovery gave me back a choice I thought had been long taken away from me. I didn't always follow through when I should have. Sometimes I picked up these discoveries and put them back down again instead of applying them. Having mental health conditions at times made it hard for me to make the commitments to my health I needed to. But, like everything I have since learned about being a human, when I was more consistent with the application of what I learned, my brain actually liked it and got me thinking about it more and more, which made me interested enough to act on it more and more. Our brains need repetition for anything to stick. When I finally threw my hands in the air in frustration with myself and committed to really following through even on my worst days, *I* started to manage my health instead of always being *managed by it*. This was when self-indulgence was dropped in favor of self-care.

It was the first time I took my eyes off everyone around me and what their bodies could do, or what "being healthy" was supposed to be, and paid some attention to my own in a loving and curious way.

I started to book massages and take relaxation and stretching classes regularly instead of running, and learned to meditate and control my thoughts because I noticed that these kinds of classes and behaviors gave me energy rather than creating more fatigue that led to more pain, and managed to keep my immune system under control at the same time. I surmised that it was about making things work for me, not trying to approach it like anyone else, because my body was never going to be textbook normal. Some days I could do heaps of exercise, others I struggled to even get out of bed because of pain or fatigue, but after a while, I learned what kind of movements and activities would help me on those days that were incredibly hard. I started to see that my body had clear responses to what I did, how I did it, and when. I couldn't see it before because I was too busy just trying to survive the day and was treating my body like some dead weight I had to carry around with me while I suffered. But when I took the time to write everything down—and I mean *everything*—it was clear my body had been trying to tell me what worked for it all along!

I sometimes bit off way more than I could chew by going far too extreme far too quickly with all the things I was testing on myself. Sometimes the only way to learn is to fall flat on one's face many, many, many times until you can see the pitfalls before you fall in! I had to work out what was going to work for me mentally, emotionally, and physically. I kept my head as firmly planted in "tracking of patterns" mode as I could. I didn't know that I had stumbled into mindfulness and self-care. And I certainly didn't realize that all of this fit under the banner of *wellness*. All I knew was that it was beginning to work and I wanted more of it.

I started to see the human form as a system of physical, mental, and emotional alignment. So I broke that down into movement, nutrition, and rest, how we think and how we express our feelings. The human body operates best when it moves, or is being moved with the assistance of others, from exercise to sex. The brain is designed to think. Humans are designed to have emotional responses and needs. Suppression of any of our needs or functions, throws the human system out of whack. It was so apparent to me at this point that there was nothing disconnected or separate in the ways this may affect life. All I could spot was a connection.

So I tested and tracked countless activities and behaviors until I found the combination that worked for me. I tried dozens of exercises, meditation, and breathing techniques, and studied the brain and body before locking into what was going to move my needle because there was no one and no information to guide me at the time. When I started actively aligning my physical, mental, and emotional systems, my life changed drastically. I was not just coping or even managing. I was now thriving. Do I still have some bad days? Yes, of course; the diseases I have are incurable. But it was like finding the accelerator when all I had ever seen was the brake in my life-car, and then getting to push down on it for the first time. The better I got, the more resilient I became. The more resilient I became, the more I realized I was living proof that it worked.

I studied my butt off and used myself every day as a test. I didn't always get it right. Many times I caused myself discomfort and emotional anguish when a type of exercise turned out to be inflammatory rather than anti-inflammatory, for example, or when I compared my body to someone else's and adjusted my behavior accordingly, something I did for way too long in my young life; but this did not deter me. The alternative was to go back to living a life ruled by pain and illness as well as housing a counterproductive mind that overflowed with resentment towards my body. That simply wasn't an option I was willing to live with anymore. I had seen the other side, and for once the grass was actually greener.

As I discovered the word *wellness*, I started to see its relationship to self-care. **Wellness is the alignment of a person's physical, emotional, and mental well-being,** effectively everything I had been discovering for myself over time. **Self-care is the delivery system that makes wellness holistic and sustainable.** It breaks those pillars of wellness down into bite-sized chunks of awesome so that people discover the exact steps they need to take to get the quality of life they desire. It is not a one-size-fits-all approach but an approach that is designed to take the unique needs of each individual into account, just like it considered my symptoms. Self-care was like a checkpoint system I could use to ensure I had actively done something for all three pillars of my wellness on any given day; and allowed me to tackle each pillar one tiny bit at a time, so I could assess what worked for me.

These patterns I saw in myself started to become obvious to me in others. When we genuinely care for ourselves in ways that suit us, not someone else, we position ourselves to harness everything we have at our disposal. This confirmed for me what I had been suspecting: wellness delivered through self-care is simply the best way to honor and amplify what we all are regardless of our complexities and idiosyncrasies—HUMAN.

When we are at our most human, we are also at our most capable. That is when we have the best shot at having the best quality of life. I wasn't looking for a cure. I was no longer interested in being whatever the fad version of *healthy* was. I didn't want to be ripped anymore. I was seeking the best possible **quality of life** I could have so that I wasn't just making it through the day, but actually getting to live the day. Self-care was a game-changer for me.

When all this clicked into place, I stopped pining for the nice-to-have situations I had wanted previously, like doing a high-impact team sport or aiming for jacked Madonna arms, and zeroed in on the stuff that actually made my life livable. I stopped asking my body to be something it was not and instead amplified what I could do by listening to my body intently and learning how to speak back to it in its own language. This is why self-care counts. It allows people to find things that they *can* sustain rather than things they *think* they should be doing but struggle to get done. The added benefit was that when I lived through wellness, I realized I had a system in place that was adaptable, that I could keep using and modifying as my body naturally did with age, something we all have to go through if we are lucky. So, even when facing new challenges, I knew exactly how to approach it. That is called having an anchor, and it is hugely helpful since change is the most inevitable, but also the most unsettling, part of being a human.

To be truly human, we must respect, develop, and *actively nurture* the connection between the physical, mental, and emotional. Absolutely everything is connected within the human body. Think of it like a car engine. If something is faulty, the rest of the engine has to take the pressure, and eventually something will give. That's how the body works too. It could be your emotional state that takes the blow, or your physical or mental health. Your job is to find out how *your* engine works and then actually work it. I used self-care to learn what kind of engine I had and how to make it run sustainably. I stopped attacking my engine with a metaphorical wrench for not working how it "should" and started applying self-care like regular car maintenance. So much of what I've achieved comes from this root.

I highly suggest you track yo'self before you attack yo'self! Get an app, open a word document, grab a diary, do some wellness coaching, get a carrier pigeon to bring you paper and pen—whatever works for you! Start by focusing on the three pillars of wellness to recognise if you are actively doing something to maintain or improve each one. Then discover what things fall into the self-indulgent category versus the self-care one by paying attention to how you feel at the time and after doing that activity or behavior. Then start eliminating the indulgent things that don't make you feel good, nourished, and capable long-term, and substitute things into your life that do make you feel that way instead (as you discover them). Sure, have some self-indulgence every now and then—hell, I am a sucker for a good shoe sale—but think more about sustainability than short-term hits of joy, and you will find that you actually respond better to that overall because that's how your body works.

If you aren't sure what to try, go totally left of field and attempt something you never would have imagined you'd agree to. Only ever weight lifted? Challenge yourself to a month of deep stretching! Only done yoga? Go to a group boxing class and shake things up. Hate talking about your feelings? Try writing down some of your feelings in a diary instead. Don't really dig the whole meditation thing? That's cool. Learn a breathing technique you can do in bed at night instead. Feel like life is a never-ending drama? I feel you. Start a gratitude diary and start discovering the tiny moments of the day that are actually decent. The answer is not identical from one person to the next. You might need help to tackle these things. Don't let the world tell you that it's 'better the devil you know'. It's not. You can't find out if there is an open-channel to all the untapped-awesome inside yourself unless you get out of your own way. This isn't to say that what you're doing is wrong or not enough (especially if you are chronically ill or disabled- it is ALWAYS ENOUGH). What I am saying, is that with finite resources at your disposal, you will want to use them where it counts for you the most.

You genuinely have nothing to lose and a hell of a lot to gain by tracking yourself even for a month. These acts of self-care, which lead you to attain your optimal wellness as you define what works for you and do those things *regularly*, will help you get the best possible outcomes in every area of your life, not just your health. So go and define *your* self-care system so you can actually enjoy your human experience!

WELLNESS TIP:
Self-Care vs. Self-Indulgence

Self-care is *sustainable* (routinely done; fits into your lifestyle; serves your mental, physical, and emotional self; and has a long-lasting effect on your well-being). Some examples are

- movement,
- meditation, and
- mantra.

Self-indulgence is based on *instant gratification* (something that is done every now and then that gives you a temporary boost but doesn't sustain long-term and is not easy to repeat regularly or can be damaging to repeat often). Some examples are

- shopping for new clothes when you feel low;
- consumption of substances like alcohol as a default response to stress; and
- binge eating.

4

GROW INTO A ROSE

Pain and illness are things we all experience in life, and they really can't be avoided. Our inclination, though, is to avoid them at all costs. Even though pain and illness are my constant companions, I have heard myself offering comfort to family and friends in times of need that directly conflicts with this undeniable fact. "I won't let anything hurt you" has fallen from my lips more than once. It sounds like a good idea to say this in the moment, and if you've found yourself uttering this line, you might even mean it at the time. But you and I both know that this is an impossibility. You will have felt pain and sickness and will again, and you can't protect yourself or anyone from them either. And this learned avoidance, or false protection from pain, does each of us a disservice in life, making us unprepared for the reality we will find.

I don't know about you, but I certainly spent a significant amount of time and energy on the pursuit of this impossible dream of no pain. I have done my darnedest to shy away from conflict with others and within myself. I've gone to great lengths to ignore it or go above it, below it, or around it, and I have tried to swallow it down or feign total ignorance of its existence. Perhaps we all have!

The terms *chronic pain* and *chronic disease* were a bit of a mystery to me even though I lived with them. I really didn't know what they would mean for me when I first heard them. I feel like the words *unrelenting* and *unforgiving* suit the situation much better. I couldn't wrap my head around the idea that I was always going to be in some level of pain or be ill more than the average person. At first, it was a soul-destroying concept, and I railed and pushed against it. I pretended. I covered up. I acted fine. I became exceptionally good at being "fine," a default for many of us with stigmatized conditions. I played drawn-out games in my mind. I did anything and everything to avoid having to confront the idea that my pain would always be there and to avoid anyone else being able to notice it. And for a long time, it seemed like a curse and created some of the lowest emotional points in my life. A considerable amount of my mental health sufferng came from the fear of the pain I had experienced and knowing I lived with a condition that could bring that on at any moment, often without a trigger. PTSD, anxiety, depression, and OCD are a diabolical combination, I can assure you. Add pain to that and it's quite the pity party!

I didn't just struggle with this concept of pain and sickness; I was utterly consumed and debilitated by it. In the very early days of my illness being recognised formally, my parents wisely decided to get a pet, hoping it would give our family unit something else to nurture besides my body. I wasn't so good at looking after myself back then, as I didn't know what to do or what steps to take. My parents got a golden Labrador we called Beau, and he was a delight. Sweet Beau heard all my troubles and gripes. I would race home after school and head to the back door knowing that his tippy-tap feet and waggy tail and the softest puppy beans on his big paws would be waiting to greet me. When I saw him, all the terror I had been through that day at school with pain, emotion, and bullying melted away. I would even climb inside his dog kennel with him, holding him tight and telling him my woes, knowing I would feel a little better once my head was buried in his warm fur near his velvet-soft ears. Dogs sense things we don't. I would be awake during the night fretting and in pain, and I would hear him walk around the outside of the house, stop outside my bedroom window, and pant gently like he was trying to say, "I am here, and I love you." I think he could genuinely tell when I was distressed. He helped me so much during that time. Beau wasn't a true service animal. He wasn't formally trained, and this was before service animals really existed for conditions like mine. But that's what he was for me, in a way.

Many years later, I began to understand chemically why pets are so brilliant. Hugging and petting them allows a release of oxytocin, our natural painkiller that can also calm emotion, and I was later able to use that discovery to help myself in other ways. Honestly, no matter what age you are, if you face unrelenting pain or illness of any kind, please consider getting a pet!

Beau helped me survive those early years of torture, and I owe some of my survival to him, but when I grew up, moved out of home and started adulting, Beau stayed behind. I realized quickly that I had to face all of this without the cuddles of a constantly molting dog and the sweet, sweet pain relief he chemically gave me on the daily. And I was bad at it for a long time. I wasn't good at talking about my situation. In fact, I was petrified to do so because I was so scared of being seen as sick or weak or damaged. I didn't know how to ask for help because when I had done that, I had been misdiagnosed and made to feel I was the cause of my own illness. Instead, I did some serious stick-my-head-in-sand action and tried to start my adult life as though none of this was happening to me. Sometimes it was for financial reasons. It ain't cheap to live if you have a lifelong illness! Sometimes it was pride, an unwillingness to acknowledge that I didn't have the necessary coping skills to manage what I was facing as a fresh adult in the big, bad world. Some of it was just that I didn't know what I didn't know, but I was about to learn!

So much of my focus was used to avoid my misery, and as a result, I was missing the biggest point of all. Even in avoidance of it, I was still giving pain my full attention! It was all I could see, feel, and experience, and it overshadowed every moment of my life, both day and night. I was focusing my mind in a purely negative direction. I thought about it, obsessed over it, felt it, and used it to create limitations in my own experience of life. *I can't do that* became a common thought in my mind if I wanted to go out or try a new experience. I had decided that pain would get in my way. And because it's all I thought about, I was reinforcing that concept in my mind over and over again. It added fuel to the fire and was making the pain stronger and the bouts of malady more regular.

My desire to distance myself from it left me steering away from all sorts of things that I now associated with pain or as a type of pain. I became the ultimate people-pleaser, never wanting to upset anyone, which led to me being a doormat and very dissatisfied. It led me to pick the wrong people to hang around with, and those people led me into all sorts of crappy experiences that only reinforced the negativity I felt towards myself, lowering my self-esteem in the process. I would do practically anything to avoid an argument and found a conflict of any kind incapacitating. I would freeze up during discussions or heated debates and become unable to produce any words from my mouth (ah, PTSD, my old friend). And often I would say or do things when I was in pain that I later couldn't remember and that I would deeply regret. When we hurt, sometimes we end up hurting others too, especially if we aren't dealing with it head-on.

This is something my amazing husband, Diesel, also had to learn to navigate among a million other things. I can't tell you how many times I have frozen up mid-discussion like a deer in headlights, but he's learned over time how to bring me out of my head and back into my body. My amazing man pays such close attention to the things I discover and share in my presentations. He learned he could help me release oxytocin and calm my sympathetic nervous system and decrease my cortisol and adrenaline levels by giving me back rubs up and down either side of my spine. He immediately started doing that without me having to ask! If I am sitting in front of a plate of food, having a serious inner battle to force-feed myself, which can happen for weeks at a time, or if I am struggling to talk about what's going on inside, he is right there next to me giving me back rubs and doing what he can to make things a little easier for me. This actually calms my cortisol receptors, which, when flared, inhibit my ability to eat well (for some people, they can stimulate them, making them want to eat anything and everything) and can cloud my judgment.

Can I just make a sidenote here and acknowledge the carers like him that truly, truly try to help and learn and actually listen to you instead of projecting their own stuff on you? Thanks, folks. They don't all consider themselves to be "carers" (my lovely man doesn't), but they end up taking on that role in many ways. Let's give them some love too. It is not easy to navigate these murky waters. My man is the best of the best, but he had to learn it all from scratch, and that wasn't always fun, I am sure!

Anyhow, I have digressed. My pain was making it hard for me to seize the day, and I am sure that, as a result, I missed out on several brilliant experiences. Unfortunately, when I realized that an opportunity might require me to learn a new skill, for example, I saw that as a type of pain and my head said, "I can't do that," so I stubbornly held my shaky ground and watched those chances fly right by me. I buckled myself into the passenger seat of my own life as opposed to the driver's seat. I became stuck, unable to advance and unable to grow. Dance became my lifeline.

Like so many other amazing lessons, I learned a crucial one on stage that has taken me years to solidify. I can't quite believe I'm going to share this with you, but here we go!

I was due to dance in a performance in a large theater, but I had been struggling with a significant amount of pain throughout my body in the week leading up to the particular day in question. I had successfully performed several times already the same week, gritting my teeth and swallowing the warning signs. Before the Thursday-night show, I was incredibly bloated and nauseated and had been unable to eat very much at all, but when it came to dancing, the old saying "The show must go on" was the credo I lived by. Rather than pulling out of the performance and letting the understudy take to the stage, I bit down hard on my inner cheeks and forced myself to show up at the venue to perform as planned.

I did my warm-up, and throughout, I was sweating bullets and the many layers of stage makeup I had applied were dripping off my face. I squeezed into my leotard, skirt, and dance shoes, an ivory-colored outfit with silver sequins adorning it, with a soft chiffon bottom layer to complete the look. At this stage, with my sweaty appearance and protruding gut, I looked ready for an ambulance ride, but I figured that I only had to perform the routine for three minutes, then I could take a breather before my next performance, and surely everything would be fine.

As I stood at the side of the stage between the back two curtains, I could feel the pre-performance adrenaline as it made its way through my body (still the most amazing feeling in the world, by the way). Right before a performance, I usually felt as if I desperately needed to pee and had gotten quite used to this feeling being my version of "normal," but on this day, I was feeling some rumblings in the jungle from an adjacent exit. I took a few deep breaths and chose to ignore it. The pain in my abdomen and throughout my body went into overdrive as the adrenalin increased my heart rate. I could barely stand up straight, but again I ignored it.

The music came on, and I started counting the beats, waiting for my cue to enter the stage. I felt atrocious, but before I knew it, my cue came, and with a "Five, six, seven, eight," I pointed my toes and took my first step onto the stage, with the adrenaline helping to give me the energy to move with grace. I plastered a smile on my face, having used the old dance trick of spreading Vaseline on my teeth so I would keep my pearly whites visible, and did my job, and I got through about half of the routine in this manner.

As I moved into center stage, preparing for my *grand jeté en tournant*, I felt an intensely hot and sharp pain stab through my abdomen and into my hip joints and thighs. It felt like all the air had suddenly been sucked out of my body. I couldn't breathe at all. I tried to move my body into "preparation position" for my aerial maneuver, and as I did, I lost control of my bowels. Yes, as I perched on one leg with the other lifted behind me in an ivory outfit, I pooped myself. In. Front. Of. An. Audience. If you're laughing right now, it's OK because I am too.

Embarrassed, shocked, and mortified, I thankfully reacted with professional instinct. I didn't run off stage. I wasn't sure if the poop had made it out of my leotard and onto the stage yet, but running didn't seem like a very wise choice. Instead, I gently crouched to the ground and used my skirt to create a bed for me to sit on. I lifted my face to the audience with a smile, and on the spot, I made up some choreography using my arms that was a vague match for the remainder of the performance.

For the next one and a half minutes—perhaps the longest of my life—I pretended that what I was doing was planned. The rest of the dancers adapted and worked the rest of the routine around me. As the performance finished, everyone exited the stage as intended, but not me. Too scared to stand up, I did a dramatic pose and beamed from ear to ear, taking in the applause and praying for the stage to swallow me whole. Like I went on to say to my own dance pupils many years later, if you are going to do something, do it gloriously!

My lips quivered, and I wrapped myself in my skirt as the curtain came down, and I awkwardly made my way off the stage. I had managed to contain the spill within my costume. I headed to the bathroom to clean myself up. I still have no idea how much the audience saw, but no one said anything to me, so perhaps I got away with it after all. Thankfully, social media wasn't a thing back then!

Not really what most would consider a "shining" moment in my past, but in reflection, I can spot the comedy in the situation. And more importantly, it taught me some very valuable things.

I had to sit on stage in my own crap, quite literally, to learn that I couldn't avoid my pain and that I needed to listen to it. It was going to be in my life whether I liked it or not. Pretending that it wasn't happening wasn't working for me at all. I had to acknowledge the truth and find a way to get through it, not over it, under it, around it, or with an "ignorance is bliss" mentality headlining my show. Going through it was the only option.

I had to learn this lesson publicly, which was quite confrontational and not at all gentle. I had to learn to cope at that moment with the situation. I had proven to myself that I couldn't pretend that my situation would not affect me from time to time. Sometimes things would go askew. And I had to reclassify the pain from being my whole existence to merely being a part of my life that I needed to work with instead of against if I ever wanted to succeed and have some semblance of happiness.

I proved to myself that crappy day (pun very much intended) just how resilient I could be. I got back up on that stage only a short time later, in a different costume of course, and performed my heart out, actively using the movement of the gorgeous contemporary routine as a way to release some of the pain and all the emotion I had just experienced, and I killed that performance! And I proved to myself that I was not weak at all, nor limited in what I could do. I was strong and courageous and very, very capable. Most other people would have just gone home, quit the business, and never returned to it, but I understood adversity and how to overcome it because by then I had years of practice. That is called strength and growth, not weakness. When we face our pain, we do a lot of growing. Equally so, at other times in my career, I learned to bow out when I had to; and while that initially felt like weakness, I soon realized it shows real courage and common sense to advocate for what you need.

I'd love to tell you that the lesson I learned on stage that day transferred across all other areas of my life immediately, but that would be a lie. It did take many years and a lot of practice to stop thinking of the pain and sickness as enemies and start considering them to be companions and trusted advisors. I now know them well, and though I may not always like what they have to say or love the moments they pick to scream at me inconveniently, they are companions who have taught, and continue to teach, me about myself, allowing me to have a stronger mindset than many people I meet. Pain and discomfort are important educators.

When you consider your own pain, whether it manifests physically, mentally, or emotionally, or in struggles at work, conflicts in your relationships, indecision in business, or low self-esteem, I can tell you this with great certainty: Sometimes you need to sit in your own crap (sometimes, less literally than I did) in order to grow. **Being present with your manifestation of pain makes the experience of it far less severe and much more useful.**

When you avoid dealing with it, you hand over control to it. I can also safely say that your pain will always look for options to come out of you and express itself. Pain has many faces and many disguises. You may break out in a rash. Perhaps you will get a migraine. Maybe you'll pick a fight with your partner over something that later seems silly. Maybe you will do something that you can't take back, no matter how much you want to. You might find yourself crying or shaking uncontrollably or scoffing down a whole tub of ice cream for breakfast. Whatever form it comes in, think of it as a voice. Pain will have its say. You can try to silence it, you can try to ignore it, but I guarantee you that it will not work.

Over the coming years, I did develop many active coping strategies for pain and sickness from a physical perspective. And I did that through self-care by defining what movements helped reduce the pain and what breathing techniques and meditation styles kept my adrenaline and cortisol at the right levels for me. But in all honesty, my mindset around pain was the hardest issue to crack and the most important (and requires regular reinforcement). Pain does a real number on the brain and body—effectively physiologically gearing us to experience even more of it. Finding ways to cope with pain is essential for survival. Pain is important, though. From a biological point of view, it is there to help draw our attention to something that is happening within; but it is not a punishment. That counts for emotional pain too! I learned over time that I would always experience pain, but I had a choice whether or not that pain caused me to suffer. That is not a physical difference but a mental one. Most people want to be distracted, to find ways to be unaware of the pain. But I have not found this to be very effective. Quite often, if pain is being ignored, it will simply find new ways to grab your attention. So if pain normally makes you snappy and you don't address it, it might throw a new symptom at you, like making you queasy, so that you pay attention to it.

People with high levels of physical pain or chronic illnesses may have brains that end up operating a bit differently. Many people with trauma also experience this. Our limbic system and amygdala just don't switch off. Our neurons are firing twenty-four hours a day, keeping our threat-perception sector running and unable to switch off. Comparatively, people who get an injury or have an awful week may feel pain, and these parts of the brain will switch on, but they will eventually calm down and work in equilibrium with the rest of the brain. If you are traumatized or chronically ill, they may stay on all the time. It is *literally* exhausting, and funnily enough, that exhaustion makes pain stronger or its reoccurrence higher, making it harder to sleep. A lack of sleep can make you so tired the pain gets worse. It's a brilliantly complex, vicious cycle. This is why people don't just "get over" things all the time. Sometimes it is about management instead of a cure.

The biggest shifts I had to make when it came to pain were not the physical ones but how I viewed the pain. I now know that ignoring it, distracting myself from it, or being angry at it or fearful of it leads me down a bad path where I effectively climb into the back seat of my own life vehicle, holding my legs to my chest while I rock back and forth with my eyes shut as Pain gets into the driver's seat and steers me wherever it wants to go, usually somewhere self-destructive and scary. So I have chosen to get to know it, to understand it, to chat with it, to learn from it, to hold its hand gently, and to allow it to guide me without ever letting it take the reins entirely. This doesn't mean I am never sad or panicked about it, I am entitled to my human reactions to such things of course, and sometimes the starting point is a solid snot-rolling-down-my-face-head-pounding-cry or meltdown, but I am quick to check in with the pain and listen to it rather than getting worked up about it. What I have learned is that when my pain feels heard, it usually stays within my means of control.

Over many years I have painted a mental image of pain—how it works and what its purpose is. We all face it. Sometimes it's long periods of mental or emotional anguish, and other times it's physical. However, few people seem to be able to actually cope with it. We aren't taught how. Like I said, the biggest lesson has been in mindset. So here is a mental image I hope will work for you no matter what kind of pain you face in life.

These days I filter the necessity of pain through the lens of a rose. A rose is a beautiful flower and one of the most favored of all the flowers in the world. Its stunning variety of petal colors and sweet aromas lead to an impact when they are given or received, evoking love, kindness, forgiveness, celebration, or empathy. In other words, this is a flower that makes an impact. However, it grows in manure. It doesn't just magically appear in its glorious form. It grows its way there through layers of soil and poop and earthworms and rain. The rose works through what we would consider to be pain to become what it is destined to be, making an impact when it does so. If it didn't, it would shrivel up and die, never producing a single gorgeous flower. And you and I will have to do the same throughout life. So when you find yourself sitting in the poop, confronted with pain, take a moment to be present with it. Don't turn away; try to go around it, above it, or over it. Go through it and grow into the unique rose you are meant to be.

WELLNESS TIP:
Change Your Pain Game

Pain is not a punishment. Pain is a communication tool and an educator. Instead of trying to avoid it or trying to battle it, try tuning in to the many things it is attempting to tell you.

If you want to grow into a rose, you will have to grow through your manure sometimes.

5

FIND PURPOSE

My bare feet are cold on the old wooden floorboards, but they reverberate with the baseline of the music, warming them and making them come alive while the kick drum and my heartbeat come into alignment. The minor-key violins pulse through me like flashes of lightning. My breathing changes as I am drawn to the percussion. I am in a different place. I am inside myself. I am present in every muscle and bone. As the music layers build, I feel the layers of my body do the same. I do not think. I just am. I allow myself to be the vessel. My shoulder rolls back, and my chest lifts to the sky. My muscles move both on the beat and within the gaps between them. The balls of my feet play with rhythm as I find the strength in my posture. I turn my head to the right, propelling my body into a fast spin, like a leaf spinning in the wind, and with the smallest adjustment in my breath and my weight shifting from the ball of my foot to the heel, I come to a graceful pause. My arms rise from the elbows upward, not angular but curved like the wings of a bird. I arch my body, leaning to the side, my face tilted to the sun. My birdlike form ready to fly. I shut my eyes for a moment to feel both lost and found. I flash my blue eyes back open and hold eye contact with myself in the mirror. There I am. I am unstoppable but vulnerable. I am expression. I am feeling. I am pain and joy and confusion and clarity. I am alive. My brain is awake, my neurons are firing. As my body soars through the air as I leap, I am transported through a tunnel of memories from the past to the present over and over again. Each journey brings me closer to understanding who I am, what I am, what I have done, what has happened to me. This is all encapsulated in a beat, in a single moment. All emotion, all pain is outside of me now, exorcised and free of my form. I land gently, feeling the gravity as it works through my knees and calf muscles. I exhale slowly, never breaking eye contact as I contract my upper back muscles towards each other to change the shape of my wings into gentle arms. I raise my body upon my feet, not simply lifting but working through every single muscle, until I can be no taller. I find my center, and there I hold, suspended in this state of powerful presence.

Dance, moving the body, channeling music, and not having to use words is such an incredible thing. Not everyone is a born dancer, but we all have something if we search for it, something that can't be replaced. So one of the trickiest moments for me to navigate came when I was told I would not be able to pursue my dream of being a professional performer because of my health. A well-meaning specialist bluntly declared that I would need to "give that up and pick something more realistic" to do with my life. In his opinion, the stress caused by doing anything physically or mentally demanding made my dream career choice a risky one. But he also told me I likely wouldn't be able to work full-time or have a business either. Many options weren't left on the table after that appointment!

I had such a strong reaction to that declaration, perhaps one of the strongest in my life. I could feel every nerve ending, every cell of my body, every organ, even the hairs on my head screaming, "No, do not take this away from me! I'd rather die." I had been dreaming about and working on building a performance career for as long as I could remember. I took detours to pay the bills when I needed to, and sometimes when I doubted that I was on the right track, but I always circled back to the dream of the stage. It was in my DNA, and it was a life force that attracted me magnetically, powerfully, and was as essential to me as oxygen.

The first time I recall thinking about being a professional performer properly, though I had been on stage and loved it even as a child, was when my family and I went to see *Les Misérables*. I think I was still in primary school at the time, and it was certainly before I donned my cape of invisibility. I remember sitting in the theater in the big, soft, plush red chairs and being so close to the stage that I could see the sweat drip off the performers' bodies and spit launch from their mouths as they sang. I was captivated by every single thing that was taking place in front of me on the slowly revolving stage. When I think about it even now, I can feel the excitement that I felt then, the hairs standing up on the back of my neck, my racing heart, my shallow breaths. I remember that all I could think was, *That is what I want to do.*

It felt like most of what I'd done from that point on was gearing me in the direction of the stage. I was a decent singer and musician, having been accepted into a specialist music program in which I went to high school to learn to read and write music and play the clarinet while I was still a primary school aged child, and I was a solid actor, which I also pursued seriously for some time; but dance was where I could tell that I shone brightly. And as you know by now, it became *the* way for me to express my physical and emotional issues when words seemed to fail me. So the idea of not being able to follow my dream was unimaginable. I am so serious about this being a part of me that I have a tattoo that reads, "In music, I find hope. In dance, I find freedom." Still accurate.

The truth is, I didn't tell anyone what that physician had told me. I kept that to myself in fear that people around me would agree with him and force me out of the dance industry. Competition in the industry is very high at times. There are so many people aiming to get one of the few roles being offered. I didn't want there to be an excuse for anyone to overlook me as a prime candidate. I didn't want to be the poster child of illness. In part, I just didn't want to have to keep explaining and defending myself. I'd had a lifetime of that already, and it was exhausting and undermined my mental health too much to have to do it often. I just knew dancing was what I needed to do even if it made no sense to anyone else, so I kept my mouth shut and did it.

Dancing was one of the only things that made me feel alive, and if it had the power to make living with the disease better, even just the tiniest bit better, then surely there was something to be learned from that! Surely there was a pot of gold at the end of that double-jazz-hands dance rainbow. I was determined to find it.

As I chose to defy "authority" (how we all perceive medical professionals), I was also choosing to place a high level of importance on finding the best ways to function and achieve my goals at the same time. It was a lot of pressure, and it forced me to pay much closer attention to myself. Through the process of starting to define my self-care, I was rooting down, down, down into the rabbit hole to find any and all discoveries that might help me live the way I believed I deserved to. I was watching and noting down everything I possibly could about myself. This was not a surface-level venture, this was me out in the dark, stumbling and reaching and in among the falls finding my "eureka" moments. I noticed that I responded well, both physically and mentally, when I was performing or practicing contemporary dance, ballet, jazz, and Broadway jazz. I did much better there than I did when I was jumping into hip-hop and acrobatics routines. I would feel better longer and my muscles seemed to recover more quickly with flowing movement as opposed to more staccato movement. And because my body felt better, I also felt more evenly keeled mentally and emotionally. My immune system was better, and my pain levels were more controllable when I was flowing. I reduced the amount of hip-hop and acrobatics I did to the bare minimum and increased the rest.

Through ballet, I was inadvertently building great athletic strength and great mental and emotional discipline. Ballet reinforced the importance of foundational knowledge and why it is good to revisit the basics of anything you have learned to do in life, no matter how advanced you may think your skills are. Stability in the foundation was everything.

Ballet and jazz came with a clear set of rules and structures, and within those, my ambitions grew. I was developing a dedicated work ethic because these art forms require nothing short of total commitment. I was also learning about core strength and how many of the supporting muscles attached to the core work in unison to create a protective layer for so many areas of the body. As someone with an unstable tummy, knowing that my core was doing a good protective job was a big deal to me (it really should be for anyone).

But through contemporary dance, I learned to break and bend the rules. I was able to play with structure and learned to blend and fuse movements that wouldn't traditionally match. Contemporary dance is a true mind-body workout, with the mental, physical, and emotional working in conjunction to look effortless and emotive. I fell deeply, head over heels in love with contemporary dance because of how I felt when I was doing it and afterward. I learned that dancing is one of the best ways to access sentimental memory. When this part of the brain is switched on, our body and brain seem to function differently. We tend to be happier because we have happy chemicals in our body, like serotonin, and the body is receiving green lights from the brain to detox, fight, and recover to function at maximum capacity. This is why dance is so often used as a form of exercise for those with memory difficulties like Alzheimer's and dementia, and why it is part of my own business today where I help people with needs similar to mine. I even weave this discovery into the work I do as a keynote speaker where I pick specific music, and often encourage audiences to bust a move in any way they can, if they are able to, so they can experience the change within their brain and body in real time. When people move, especially with music, they can remember and do things they wouldn't normally be able to do. This is because music also boosts brain chemicals. Ever wonder why many physiological activities, like a workout are easier with music and much, much harder without? Now you know! This explains in part why I find dance so powerful. My pain, my mushy thinking, my volatile immune system all change when I have those parts of the brain, and the neurotransmitters that go along with the process, online.

I became deeply dialed into my physical self. I was able to spot potential injuries before they occurred, and learned how far I could push my body before my immune system set off red flags, something to be mighty aware of when your condition can cause your body to attack itself. I began to understand what kinds of pain responses meant "Today is a pajama day; don't even bother" versus "Stop everything right now; you need a breather" versus "You can keep going, but you need to move that differently."

I was manipulating my hormones and chemicals by doing certain kinds of movements at certain times, which proved to be a powerful skill to have concerning my pain. I learned that I have a window of time when pain strikes that usually allows me to take back control if I take care of my mental, emotional, and physical in that time slot. It may not eradicate all of the pain, but it positions me to be able to deal with it and usually reduce it. I was effectively creating my own natural pain relief through flowing movement by releasing endorphins, serotonin, and oxytocin. And I was controlling my cortisol and adrenaline at the same time, which can be triggered when in physical or emotional pain.

Underlying it all was the power of the breath and the way that I thought. Long before I understood it scientifically and logically, I was using a form of meditative movement on myself. Meditation and deep breathing can assist us in releasing serotonin and enhancing the effectiveness of any movement that we do alongside it. I began to approach my body with curiosity instead of fear. That curiosity grew into passion when I began to teach others to get more out of themselves through performance by using what I had been learning. In classes, I would encourage dancers to dedicate themselves to not just "marking out" a routine, but actually practicing as though they were live on stage so they could truly understand the best places to inhale and exhale in a routine. The added benefit being that, when under pressure, people revert to their most practiced state. So when the nerves kicked in, my artists knew what to do and how to do it in the safest way possible, allowing them to recover faster.

I was teaching them that they could use the breath for added power and energy, emotional output, or to find more elongation and stretch within the lines of their bodies or a specific group of muscles. I was teaching them to sustain, not just perform. I was teaching them to thrive rather than burn out. I was teaching what I had started to learn: when we connect the mind to the body, using the breath as a conduit, the body is capable of significantly more than we think. I was accessing my full human. It is through this level of connection we can manipulate our own chemical reactions. When one faces pain and illness, understanding that your body and brain are like a chemical highway and, more importantly, learning what movements and breathing patterns make your highway a great place to take a drive counts in a huge way!

It may not be much of a surprise to you that, with all of this rudimentary lived experience under my belt gained from being a dancer and having a disease, I found my way into the wellness industry. It might not be a shock that researching and finding out about my hormones and chemicals, what the breath did for the body, how my brain functioned when I danced, and more, led me to have the exact kind of knowledge to succeed in the wellness industry or to help people just like me feel hope. I didn't see at the time that all these lessons I got by sticking to my guns and chasing my dance dream had larger implications than I had intended. Knowing how to break and bend rules, learning how to align all of myself to be a good dancer, questioning the status quo by being an artist, and the level of dedication I had to make my life better positioned me to do a considerable amount more within wellness than I was ever going to be able to do with dance alone. My initial passion was dancing, but my interest in the human form was starting to match and even surpass that passion.

Wellness was a slow discovery, but one that woke me up in every way. It made me a significantly better performer, choreographer, and teacher. It made me a better person. It made my life functional. I was already investing in the physical, mental, and emotional connection of the human form. I was creating my self-care system. I was well and truly paving my own path, defiantly, stubbornly, and hopefully. I just didn't have the detailed formal education to go with it, a more rounded knowledge of what I and the rest of us deal with—our mysterious skinsuit!

Over the years, I cannot tell you the number of times health professionals have been surprised that I have been able to do so much with my body that I "shouldn't be able to." I was reporting less reliance on antibiotics to get me through bouts of sickness, I was having fewer issues controlling my OCD, and I was spending days instead of weeks in bed with pain and fatigue. It was the first time in my adult life I got to live some version of a functional life. I am glad to say that more research is being done, and more and more physicians are now embracing wellness as one of the ways people can live a better quality of life. Some physicians are becoming more open-minded about holistic health in general. They are starting to see that it's what makes the patient feel better, not what they think of it, that counts. They are getting better training on how to deal with invisible illness and chronic pain. Some places even have meditation classes on the ward! It's a snaillike pace of change, though, and the gap between the lived experience of diseases and what the medical professionals are taught is pretty mammoth.

Back then, I hadn't come across one doctor who thought what I was doing made any sense at all. I have been laughed at, had eyes rolled at me, and been told I was making a huge mistake by more than one physician, and plenty of everyday people too.

Sidenote: if you have medical issues and do not like the bedside manners of your assigned team, change them. The right people for you are out there. You should never have to defend yourself or be made to feel bad for what you face or how you are coping. And I mean that at any age. If you are young, your voice *does* count. Keep speaking your truth till someone listens. If you find yourself feeling shut down by your medical team, get a new one. I know that it feels intimidating to have to fire your doctor, but if your accountant or electrician made you feel shamed or "less than" or rolled their eyes at you, you'd fire them! That's how I had to think of it. You frankly don't have time or energy to waste on people who make you feel like that when you already face so much. I don't work with anyone these days that isn't willing to work collaboratively with me and, at times, other professionals on my team regarding my health. If they make my experience worse, I send them right out of my life, and quickly. I now have a fantastic team, including both holistic and Western doctors. Your dream team is also out there. And if you struck gold with the best team ever upfront, I am super excited for you! Celebrate that situation daily!

Sidenote aside, feeling it was all I had left, I became so dedicated to keeping my dance dream alive, that I channelled all my defiance, fear, curiosity, joy and passion into the pursuit. I pulled myself out of the hopeless pit of despair I had been buried in, and by doing so, I discovered that dance was not the only thing I was here to do at all! It was merely the catalyst that drove me to get everything I wanted, by using everything at my disposal. There is nothing that differentiates me from anyone else facing an obstacle in life, really. I have struggled hard and sometimes ended up in tears, utterly frustrated by my lack of success or inability to figure things out. I don't want to paint you a picture that says everything is perfect because that is unrealistic—I do have incurable diseases after all. I have days where I am too tired and sick to do much, so my life revolves around a mountain of dry shampoo, hours of meditation, and a lot of stretching. There are days when getting out of my pajamas, washing my face, or making a bite to eat takes every ounce of my willpower and skill. Having chronic illnesses, mental health illnesses, and pain is no joke. But by being persistent and open-minded, I have been able to take a truly awful moment in time for me and prevent it from being an obstacle to joy.

What's more important, I have used it to find tools I can use to ensure it's only *days* of dry shampoo I have to deal with instead of *weeks* of it at a time. When the going got tough, I didn't get tougher or work harder, I worked smarter. I lifted my bitter, scared, resentful head up and paid attention instead of burying myself in the declarations of others. I decided not to let myself drown, when there were times it would have been incredibly simple just to let myself sink under. I have nearly done so many times from the fatigue alone.

Please don't think I have some sort of superhuman motivation key that bolsters me in the storm; I really don't. I get grumpy, disheartened, frustrated, and sad that I don't ever get to have a day off from pain or illness. I have given blood, sweat, and tears to the pursuit of betterment. I have certainly sidestepped on the path, taken a few detours, and even done a lot of eggbeaters where I just don't seem to get anywhere, but I have always stuck it out and found a way, or found my way back to it. When I faced my worst moment, I sort of faced my mortality too. I realized this was it—this life was all I was going to get, that this body was all I was going to get. No one could make this easier for me but me. I really had nothing much left to lose, so I chased hope, determined that if I was going to go out, I was going to do so on my own terms, knowing I had given it everything I had. And by bluntly staring that obstacle in the face and forcefully telling it to move out of my way, I started an inner voyage that led me from dance into understanding the human body and mind, inadvertently into wellness and eventually into my purpose. I teach people how to understand and embrace their humanness to help them get everything they want—a good quality of life, a career, a business, relationships—the full spectrum. Because it is all connected.

My worst life moment was really my best one in disguise. It presented as a horrifying obstacle set out to destroy my only hope, my last thread and lifeline to keep me in this world; but instead, it took me on a long, winding, and profoundly personal journey. I dropped the precious attitude I had about what I thought I "should" be and started facing reality head-on. Accepting that I was never going to have someone else's "normal" day came from walking this path. Acceptance isn't giving up, it is not resignation, it is not failure. It is growth. And I honestly wouldn't have grown had I not kept following the path that was true to me. I stopped looking at myself as "sick" because that made me feel incapable of living, and I started working out what I could do with my body and mind. I stopped working to live like everyone else and started making life work for *me*.

Was it easy? No. It was exceptionally challenging because I didn't have anyone to learn from directly, but it presented me with the option to find purpose. And we all need one of those to gain fulfillment. It was necessary for my survival in more ways than one. I was able to understand that what I had been living could mean something more than "pain" and "disease." It meant that I could serve others who hadn't been served before in a way that they understood, because their lived experience was similar to my own. It meant I got the opportunity to be an example to others at the starting line of their journeys, something I desperately needed when I was a teen and a responsibility that is also an honor, and one I do not take lightly. It meant I could help people appreciate their bodies and minds and help them find beauty in their own unique design no matter what they face. I get to witness people embrace their humanness, and that is a beautiful gift that makes every moment of my life worth living.

As my purpose became clear to me, my self-esteem and confidence grew. I carried with me the gifts that being a dancer gave me—discipline, emotional expression, physical understanding of my body, the ability to take the impossible and potentially make it possible—and allowed myself to go on and do things I had initially ruled out as options for my life. I lived overseas, choreographed stage shows and music videos, built a business and speaking career, grew a relationship with my incredible husband forged by what we have faced down together, and even created what you're reading right now!

It would have been so easy to have taken the other path. To have stayed in the socially-dictated unhappiness that seems so often a reality for those of us with disabilities. I could've picked the stable options and had a calmer, more traditional life that's not a reflection of who I am and was not my purpose at all. In all honesty, even the "normal" path would not have granted me an easier time. I would have been miserable, and that would've led me to even more pain and illness. I didn't want to live a risk-averse life. I know, had I chosen that path, I likely wouldn't have done half the things I have done. I believe I would actually be much more unwell and much less happy as a person had I done what I was told and ignored what was calling to me. With my diagnosis, I was offered a way to *exist*, but I wanted a way to *live*. I listened with bated breath to my own shaky inner voice and overcame the confident, blunt declaration of someone else to get here. It is the most logically illogical sounding thing, but it was exactly what I was meant to do, and I knew that deep down inside.

I know that we all don't want the same things, but I know we do all face moments in life that are the lowest of the low, and if we let them, they have the power to attach darkness to every corner of our lives like some kind of tentacled monster connecting to a host. In these moments, we can choose to play it safe, or we can choose to leap and learn. That doesn't mean you have to fight all the time. I want to be clear: it is perfectly human to cry, to decide today is too hard, to put something off to tomorrow. Sometimes that is what you need to do, and it's OK.

Believe me, I get it! I am not saying to throw all caution to the wind. You have to do what is right for you. Deep down in your gut, in the fiber of your being, you know what is right, just as I did. However, I suggest that there is much to be gained by taking a leap and hoping that a branch is there to catch you if you fall. If you land safely, you will have gathered a lesson in faith. If you fall, as you pick yourself up off the ground, a little bruised and scratched, there are lessons to be learned there too. As you recover and recalculate your leap, you will do better next time. The scratches will heal, and you will have a neat little scar to remind you of your ability to show courage and your ability to recover from the knock-backs that come your way. And no matter the outcome of the leap, as you do this more and more, you will uncover things about yourself that might just add up to your individual purpose.

For a while there, things were petrifyingly dark for me, and while I listened to my inner voice and walked my path, there was a gnawing feeling the whole time that maybe I had got it all wrong too. I took that leap and hoped to find a branch underneath me. When the doctor told me to find something else, I just couldn't accept it. I honestly don't know if I would have survived. My defiance helped me light my way forward. But I thought I was simply step-ball-changing my life in the direction of dance, carrying the tiniest of lights with me as I did so. Low and behold, that gave me the opportunity and the motivation to dig deeper. In doing so, suddenly there was a whole other career, a whole other industry, a whole other life waiting for me. Suddenly there was a way I could help, I could serve. Suddenly there was a way for all of this anguish to have meaning. I could never have predicted that my trying to stay well enough to teach a dance class would lead me to speaking on stage about wellness or writing this book or building a business out of it. **Purpose is often there, in the rubble of our dreams.**

So when things are at their darkest, please know there is always a flicker of light. It's going to be up to you to breathe oxygen on that tiny flame to ignite a roaring fire. But when you do, it will illuminate a path just for you that you probably never knew was there.

WELLNESS TIP:
What Moves You?

There is no one type of exercise that elevates us all. Many people with chronic pain or illness face a higher inflammation index in their bodies, which means that higher-intensity workouts may hinder rather than assist day-to-day functioning, but there is a spectrum where your own personal exploration is needed. Depending on your needs, you may require the physical assistance of others or aid items to discover what gives you access to the appropriate balance within your physical systems.

My key advice is to do or participate in, movements (with or without assistance, as required) that help you to find more space within yourself. If you don't yet understand what that means, you haven't found the right type of movement yet. Keep looking, it really is out there.

6

KNOW YOUR REAL ESTATE

For three years, back in my Skrillex-haircut days, my husband and I lived in quite an old, poorly maintained apartment in one of the most popular locations in Melbourne, Australia. Being very young and both independently chasing creative pursuits (he's an incredibly talented designer and entrepreneur), we were living paycheck to paycheck but wanted to be close to our friends, great cafés, nightclubs, and the thriving dance industry hub. So we had given the apartment a brief once-over, ignoring the apartment's shortcomings, and signed on the dotted line. Voila! We had a place to live!

When we picked up our keys, we were also handed a standard lease booklet, a template used on just about every property available for rent. It included limited information like who to contact in case of a plumbing emergency and the bank details of where we should deposit our monthly rental fees. Nothing in the paperwork was what could be referred to as "useful" or "explanatory" in how to approach living in that specific property.

Let me paint a picture for you of what we were living in. A one-bedroom apartment with a tiny lounge room and an even tinier kitchen. The kitchen was so small that I could barely do a full 360-degree turn in it, and I am five foot one and petite. We had a combined bathroom and toilet with a broken exhaust fan, mold on the ceiling, and no space for laundry facilities. The carpets were dark brown with ripped patches, worn away by years of use and abuse. The bathroom and kitchen had mustard-yellow linoleum flooring. The bath, vanity unit, and toilet were the ones that came with the property when it was built in the sixties—pink and rusted. Someone had repainted the walls from baby pink to cream, splashing it on with artistic abandon in thick coats that flaked and bubbled as they dried. In fact, they had even managed to paint over the doors, door frames, handles, and mechanisms, making it impossible to shut the doors. If we wanted privacy, we had to wedge the doors closed. On windy nights we would shove socks under the wedged bedroom door to ensure it didn't fly open, and I don't think a single week went by when we lived there that I didn't find myself vacuuming up cream paint flakes.

The oven that came with the kitchen also appeared to be as old as the property itself. Australia stopped using the Fahrenheit system and switched to Celsius in 1970, and this oven was still in Fahrenheit, which was pretty shocking to me. I had never seen an oven that was in Fahrenheit before. They had all been replaced years ago! And because I had never seen one that old, I literally didn't know how to use it. I did a bit of head-scratching before realizing that, in order to heat the oven up, I had to follow a process. I needed to turn on the gas, then open the oven door, put a lighter or lit match in my hand, and fully extend my arm to the back of the oven, where the gas entered through a small opening, to ignite the gas into a flame. It took forever to get the oven to the desired temperature and even longer to cook anything in it. Let me tell you, trying to roast a chicken in that oven was an arduous, lengthy, and very hot procedure! The heat the oven produced in the apartment was a real bummer in the Australian summer, but a lifesaver in winter when it served as more of a heater than a food-preparation unit!

Not one of the things I've just described to you was contained within the lease paperwork when we received the keys. There was no manual provided for this property, and when we moved into it, it was far from an ideal design. But bit by bit over three years, we learned all of its idiosyncrasies, adjusted what we could, and even managed to get a new toilet installed (an adventure that saw me peeing in a bucket when it stopped working, and having to stay at a friend's house for a couple of nights while my lazy landlord got around to fixing it—honestly, sometimes life is just a comedy sketch in which we play the fall guy!). But the point is that we paid attention to what we were living in, put in the time to understand it, and adapted to our environment.

In many ways going from a fully functional body to one that didn't seem to comply with standard rules and formulas was a little like waking up in an apartment that I didn't recognize. It was a bit of a mess and came with no instructions. No one could tell me how to live inside this body of mine. It was left up to me to work it all out.

I've always found it exceptionally odd that, as humans, we really don't get educated on what we are, how we work, and how to get the best out of ourselves, something I believe we need to urgently rectify. Most of us spend a decade or more learning to read and write and do calculations, and learning right from wrong. We learn interpersonal skills and social norms at school, and we might even learn one or two things about exercise by participating in sports. But our focus is on preparing ourselves for a career and very little else. It's bizarre that, as a world, we're confronted with mental and physical health issues that continue to get worse, yet we don't teach kids and adults alike how to function as a human being nor how important it is to become self-aware and self-accepting instead of comparing our bodies and minds to other people's! If you end up also facing some form of condition, either physical or mental, as your life's journey progresses, it becomes even more complex to ascertain how to live than it is for the average person.

Living in that rundown apartment was fraught with complexity because so many little things didn't function as they should have. I recall standing in the kitchen one evening facing the kitchen sink, my body side-on to the oven, which only moments before I had turned on to preheat it to cook dinner. Out of nowhere, I heard this loud bang, took a hard hit to my left leg, and was slammed into the sidewall. I screamed out a couple of shocking obscenities and frantically looked down at my leg to see if I was bleeding. I wasn't—thankfully, I was wearing knee-high boots at the time—but my heart was racing anyway. I quickly realized what had happened. The base of the oven door had blown off and into my leg! It turned out that there was a fault in the gas line, and when I had lit the oven, the pressure built up inside and blew the base of the door right off. Needless to say, the oven required repairs, and I certainly had to change my dinner plans!

I think that most of us go through life like an oven with a potentially dangerous flaw, just waiting to explode. And the issue is that we wait for our oven door to fly off before we pay attention to what's going on inside our bodies and minds. We aren't taught the value and importance of what we are living in from an early age. We don't know what we don't know. And when it comes to health or mindset, having to learn everything from scratch amid trauma is extraordinarily hard. I know because I did it. I'd been handed information that was about as vague as my lease after my diagnosis. Knowing that I was going to face "digestive issues, constipation, and diarrhea" told me nothing about how to operate in a body like that, and the list of what I faced ended up being so much more extensive than what I was told. It was a long, trying journey to obtain the knowledge I needed to build a metaphorical operating manual for my body and mind.

So much will change in your life. Hairstyles, jobs, vehicles, clothing, financial stability, and more will evolve and fluctuate. The one true constant is you. You can't trade in your mind or body for a new one. Your body, your mind, and your resulting humanness equate to the *one piece of property you'll always own*. It is your forever home, and right now you might not have a clue how to live inside it. And if you don't know how to live in it now, you might be in for a rude awakening every decade or so when your body changes in huge ways again and again. You are living inside something that evolves, changes, and decays with time, and that is perfectly natural and intentional. What is normal now might not be normal for you in five or ten years. Your hormones change regularly no matter what sex you are, and your metabolism changes. Therefore, your hair, skin, mood, weight, energy, bones, and more will also change. Change happens, but how you react to those changes matters more than the change itself! And having a process that helps you understand what you are living in now will provide you with a default way to learn what you are living in when the next wave of changes carries the old you away.

When change happens, you cannot get "back to normal." That normal, that version of you, will be gone, and what is left is the process of grieving the old you, then creating a new normal for the new you. This process is utterly human, and you will need to do it repetitively throughout life. I believe that grieving happens a lot more than we acknowledge and is a bittersweet aspect of the human experience. So much of life is learning to accept our personal situations and the form we are in. I don't think it is a coincidence that the final stage of grieving is acceptance. It is part of what we do again and again to get there. Embrace it.

Having some basic understanding of how to keep your organs functioning well through movement, rest, and nutrition; how to eradicate thought patterns that undermine your efforts; and how to cope with unexpected stress will create a foundation on which you can build a stable home. When we live life as though we've walked into our home not knowing where the light switches are located, at some stage we're going to trip over something or walk face-first into a wall. Ouch! And if you don't do something about that now, the reality is that you may have to do a few more face-first wall crashes to figure it out on your path. Save yourself the heartache (and the bruises on your lovely face) by working some things out now. Believe me, it will make the next wave of change a bit easier to cope with!

Your forever home is *never* perfect. Perfection doesn't exist. Even when you buy a house, there will be things about it that frustrate you from time to time. Maybe your forever home has a few cracked tiles or faulty wiring that causes blown fuses on occasion, but wouldn't you rather know how to make the property work for you rather than feel like it's operating against you? When you don't know how it works, you will feel betrayed when it changes, and likely find yourself comparing your home against someone else's. You cannot trust something you have never bothered to get to know. Do you immediately trust strangers when you meet them on the street? No. But most of us know about as much about our forever homes as we do about strangers. Trust comes from knowledge and time and a willingness to acknowledge things as they are, not what they are compared to something else.

You can't fix everything; every property has its issues. That's not what this is about. There is no cure for the lived human experience because it is supposed to be inclusive of the black, white, and grey; the good, the so-so, and the bad; the ups, the plateaus, and the downs. But knowing the faults in your home allows you to find the things that work well, too, and gives you the chance to optimize and appreciate them. It isn't all about identifying things that don't work. Honestly, finding what doesn't work is easy since our brains are geared for survival and risk assessment. Your brain will identify the risks you face in your property design without you trying very hard. But you need to manually look for and make room for the good. You need to take the time to find it, revel in it, and use it.

When you spot the bad, take a second to find the good. It is right there inside you. Initially, it may not seem "good." If you are well down the rabbit hole of self-loathing, it may be a case of finding something that is "passable" or "OK." It takes time to fall head over heels in love with what you have with you and within you. You cannot appreciate the good things if you never bother to identify them. No matter what shape, size, or design you seem to be or what issues come with your property, there are good things waiting to be discovered! Your metaphorical bedroom might be a structural mess, but by noticing that, you might also see that your living room is your favorite space, fully loaded with surround sound, plush chairs, and gorgeous curtains.

Some people are geared to write things down, and if that's you, then start getting to know the ins and outs of your forever home and commit it to paper. But you don't have to; some people prefer to internalize and analyze. I have found that part of learning to appreciate the good things alongside the bad is to have gratitude for my body and mind. And I have done this in part by having a gratitude journal and gratitude mantra. Even on my worst, most shocking, I-have-not-left-the-bathroom-for-six-straight-hours-and-I-look-like-a-drowned-rat days, I make a point of finding something about myself I am grateful for, and I either write it down or say it out loud to myself. Gratitude actually changes the way the brain operates and thus effectively reconditions your body to be calmer and more functional. So however you do it, it is worth the effort to pay some attention to the thing that *facilitates your entire life* so you can appreciate what it is you're dealing with.

Did my "manual" identify dozens of not-so-great things about my piece of property? Sure it did. But it also helped me appreciate the things that *did* work well and the things I liked, like my eyes that operate like a mood and health ring, changing shades of blue depending on what is going on. I love my eyes now, and I draw attention to them as one of my favorite features. But initially, when I looked in the mirror, I didn't even see my eyes; I was too busy noticing how dull and sick my skin looked and how I didn't look like a "normal, healthy person." Taking a step back and working it all out helped me identify the things that were right in front of me that I had failed to notice before, and those things sometimes help me get through those super-crappy days.

On those days when I am stuck in the toilet for hours on end, I think to myself, *Bummer that it's a toilet day today, but damn, my eyes are telling a very sparkly story, and I am so grateful to have these baby blues!* On those days when I am in pain and find myself being drawn to criticize this mighty body of mine, to make mountains out of molehills, because I have acne or my weight has changed, or because my muscle has wasted away a little, I now have things I can identify about myself that I love enough to help me cope and keep those negative tapes in my mind quiet. It requires regular reinforcement, but I know it is a tool I can use, and it really does help.

You can be told by others a million times that you are pretty just as you are, or strong, but unless you actually recognize your beauty and strength from within, not just on the outside, nothing will change. With the world around me constantly projecting images of health and beauty and power that I will never be, it is easy for me to get suckered back into thinking I am not enough. But when I can say, "Flic, consider how much faster you get through your flare-ups now. You are so enough; you are doing so well," or "You're still here, Flic, even after all this, you are still here," I can recognize that my forever home is great just as it is, with all its quirks. You will do the same with the things you find about yourself. Your manual may show a hefty list of things you don't love, but you will find things you do love through the process too. Will your manual save your ass and help you cope with life's inevitable changes? Absolutely! Will it help you start the process of loving yourself? With all my heart, I fundamentally believe that it will.

WELLNESS TIP:
Your Manual

Every property has an interior and an exterior. What do you know about yours? Take a moment to identify what your property is.

Exterior:
- What are the things that function really well?
- What metaphorical "windows that stick" do you have?

Interior:
- What are the quirks of your design that you find yourself working around (like a metaphorical power point that is slightly out of reach)?
- What are the structures of your building that have proven to be helpful to have?

Take the mystery out of what you are living in and optimize its strengths!

7

RESTRICTIONS: NO. BOUNDARIES: YES!

I am not great with restrictions. When I am restricted, I feel like I am being placed inside a locked box and the walls are rapidly closing in on me. When I am restricted, it feels like something inside me is struggling to breathe. It's as though my soul is crying out for help. I become frustrated and angry, and it is a massive energy sucker. And I know I am not alone in this reaction.

When I am in that box, I don't stop, allowing the walls to close while the air is squeezed out of me, but I also don't scramble to find an exit. In the many boxes I have been placed in over my lifetime, you wouldn't find scratch marks from where I rapidly tried to claw my way to freedom. No, when I find myself in the box of restriction, and I see those walls start to close in around me, I raise my arms, press my child-sized hands on the ceiling, and check to see if it has any give. Then I lower my arms, take a breath, and stamp my dancer's feet against the floor, checking for weaknesses. I raise my arms to my sides and use my fingertips to check the sidewalls of the box for edges, idiosyncrasies, and flexibility. I take note of everything I find, and when I have discovered something that might release the pressure in the box or change its shape, I push against it.

I push gently at first, then a little harder, and then harder again until I find the exact spot in the box that is going to give the most. Once I have located it, I shift my focus and its inherent energy towards bending the walls of the box and push them farther back to give myself breathing room. I bend the box to suit me.

I am positive that I am not alone in stating that restrictions suck. Restrictions get a big fat NO from me. I don't like them, and I don't think they are useful tools in life.

Along with my condition came a whole list of restrictions, one of the biggest being food. Trying to work out what I could eat, and in what way, was a painful process, often literally. Having to face the restriction over and over again was exhausting. Long before it was considered big business or popular to offer food for people with dietary requirements (and now with a huge price tag attached, sigh), I had to walk the aisles of the supermarket with my mother, both of us picking up boxes and reading ingredients and placing them back on the shelf. Feeding me out of a package or can was no easy task because so many of the things I struggled with were used in everything from cereals to sauces, from cakes to bottled drinks. Back then, the term *gluten-free* just didn't exist in my hometown. And my allergies go far deeper than those most obvious ones like gluten too. The list of what I can't have is exceptionally long.

My condition also meant that I had to spend time working out the difference between what I was allergic to and what I was intolerant of. I had to learn what items meant, "Don't you dare even think about it," (allergies) and what meant, "You can have a bite or two" (intolerances). I had to learn the hard way that intolerances were cumulative in my system, so "You can have a bite or two" didn't mean daily or even every second day. If I consumed my intolerances regularly, the inflammation in my body would build up over time until I would end up flared up and miserable for days or even weeks.

Some foods I could eat, but only if cooked, mashed, or pureed. Raw foods were and can still be very hard for me to digest at the best of times. Allergic reactions could set in from food in under twenty minutes and could result in a lot of pain, rapid weight loss (this is not a good thing; do not ever wish for rapid weight loss), and emotional upset for me, sometimes for a month or more. The gut is not a fast healer! I also learned that, once I was in a full flare-up state, my immune system would also suffer, bottoming out quickly or sometimes attacking me. Often, what started as a flare-up or reaction to food would also result in me getting a cold, sore throat, or virus, and my mental health would plummet alongside all of that. And a reaction from IBS could trigger Crohn's and vice versa. If I was inflamed, I was also more prone to severe fatigue, not just "I am tired" fatigue, but feeling like it was beyond my capability to lift my arms above my head. The fatigue often resulted in further pain and the inability to sleep, which would then lead to more pain, compromised immunity, and psychological issues. While food was not the only trigger for these things, it was one of the largest and most complex to understand.

Given that I was barely a teenager as this journey began, I felt like I was living in a constant state of FOMO, or fear of missing out. Every day, I watched the other kids eating their pastries and chocolates, drinking juice boxes, and enjoying the packaged foods everyone loves. I would sit with my friends, eating my cold brown rice, broccoli, and pumpkin and try to fake being excited to eat essentially the same thing every day. I hated it, and it started to rub off on how I was feeling about my body and my life in general.

I can safely say in reflection that, despite that, I was exceptionally blessed. I was blessed with a mother who continued to try foods and search for things I could eat, and she did this for a sullen and miserable teen. Mum, you're a saint! I was exposed to a lot of cooking growing up. All of the matriarchs in my family—Mum, Nana, and Granny—were excellent cooks, and I spent a lot of time in the kitchen with them. These phenomenal women would take ingredients and create food that did much more than satisfy hunger. What they cooked wasn't merely a meal. It was nourishment. It was love. It was strategy. It was nutrition. Frankly, some of it was art (my mum's lemon meringue pie, for example, is a masterpiece). They took financial restrictions, ingredient restrictions, time restrictions, and more and turned them into boundaries to operate within, transforming the ingredients into something that unified, healed, and fueled us as a family. I had role models, folks, no doubt about it.

In the kitchen, I was encouraged to be hands-on. I was grating, mixing, rolling, cutting, and licking the cake batter off the wooden spoon from a very young age. So when I was faced with a life where food could equal pain and illness, I had experience to fall back on to help me cope. It didn't feel that way initially because I was young, full of hormones, and feeling very sorry for myself. It took some time to stop looking at the walls of the box closing in on me and start doing something about it.

On occasion, my mum worked late into the evening, and though she would have prepared the bulk of the meal ahead of time, on those evenings, my sister or I was tasked with completing the meal and serving the family. That might mean preparing a side serve of veggies or cooking some rice or pasta, for example. That was the inspiration I needed to get me to start putting my arms up to the ceiling of that box of restriction I found myself in.

For many months I would cut up broccoli and microwave the dishes Mum had pre-cooked for us so that I could serve dinner to the family. And I did it with gritted teeth, and often a toxic attitude that I pushed on to those around me. I could be hurtful to others with my words if someone crossed my path when I was feeling restricted and unwell. The last thing I wanted to do was look at food, especially if I was nauseated, let alone have to serve it up to others. But I didn't back away from the task, and as I kept at it, I became less suffocated by it. And the less suffocated I was about it, the less toxic I became to be around. Instead of the walls closing in, I was starting to find the edges of the box walls. I'd task myself with finding ways to change what I was doing with the limited ingredients I could have, such as overcooking the broccoli to make it softer, adding black pepper for flavor, and attempting to make fluffy mashed potatoes without adding margarine.

This continued into the summer school holidays, when I would spend a week or so with my granny. She allowed me to cook for her and play with ingredients and the equipment in her kitchen. This gave me free rein to experiment with flavors, textures, and styles of cooking. I found ways to create desserts, which were strictly in the no-no category, that I could actually eat. My granny kindly tolerated my shenanigans, even taste-testing everything I presented to her. As she chewed whatever I put in front of her, she would look up at me with a smile and comment on everything that seemed good or right about what I had put together, while leaving out everything bad—bless her cotton socks.

Bit by bit, I was becoming more confident in my ability to cook, but more importantly, to cook for myself. I was learning to take something I was scared of and resented and turn it into something that could help fuel me in more ways than one. Each time I attempted a new dish and the outcome was a flop, that was just me checking for the edges in the box. And as I found more things I could eat, that was simply me finding ways to push against the walls of the box and bending them to fit me. I can cook a potato in more ways than I can describe!

For anyone with a food restriction, I cannot stress enough how essential this was for my progress in every way. I encourage you with all my heart to experiment and play, to find the edges of the box you've been put in and bend them to your will. Instead of being crushed as the walls close in, you will be able to push the walls away so you can breathe.

Fast-forward through two decades or so, and the lessons I learned by getting in the kitchen and changing my own situation continue to pay dividends. The lessons have been layered like a gluten-free, dairy-free, fructose-free cake, and believe me, they can actually taste good.

Food was so symbolic of how my life seemed as a teen. I was terrified of it, angry at it, and resentful that I needed it. But humans have to eat to survive, so I had to find a way around it. Three times a day, every day, I was going to be confronted by something that could make me very sick, even hospitalize me, and yet three times a day, I was going to have to eat something. But as I pushed against the walls of the restrictive box and empowered myself to try new foods or ways of preparing them, I was actually learning how to change my restriction into a boundary instead.

Going into my battle with inflammatory bowel disease, no one ever told me how much mental calculation would need to be done around food alone. While most people live meal to meal, I have had to learn to think of every meal as a gateway to how I will feel across the next few days or week and adjust accordingly. If I eat something raw, I might have to adjust my food to be soft and mushy without spice for the next three days to counter it. This is why meal prepping is a vital part of my strategy. This way, I always have a variety of nutritious meals in my freezer ready to be pulled out and used at a moment's notice depending on how my body reacts. It also helps me on those days when fatigue makes cooking way too laborious. If I have been in a public place, exposed to lots of potential germs, eating fast food isn't going to give appropriate resources to my immune system, so I have to up my nutrient density for days. And as I face issues with absorbing nutrients, I have had to work out how to get a lot more inside me at each meal than others would and use supplementation made specifically for me by a naturopath to bolster me when needed.

There is a huge amount of extra mental load, calculation, and self-awareness required to live well, but instead of seeing it all as restriction, I see it as a boundary and thrive within the parameters by paying real attention to what works for me and gearing my life to suit myself (food prepping, for example). These things may sound like a lot of work, but they save me a load of time and help me cope with the day-to-day other people don't even have to think about. If you are yet to pick up on one of my patterns, I tend to learn things and then fiff-faff about applying them to my life. So while I was learning all of this, I also struggled to advocate for what I needed when I was out or at a family function. I didn't want to be a bother or draw attention to my situation, so I would often eat things I knew would make me ill. So unrealistic. Now I don't hesitate to say what I need, and since I can cook, I will happily bring my own prepared food if needed. **Learning something is great; the application of it is what helps.**

Experimenting with food was more than just learning what to feed myself. I was also getting a crash course in inflammation, hormones, immunity function, cognitive capabilities, and endurance. As I played, I wasn't just learning recipes; I was literally adjusting the quality of my life one mouthful at a time. I was beginning to formulate a notepad in my mind on which I jotted down everything that I consumed and noted every physical, emotional, and mental reaction that I had to it in the following 24–48-hour period. As I became clearer and my mental notepad became more detailed, I was able to identify what was adding to my inflammation, what helped to reduce it, how to adjust how anxious or depressed I felt, how much longer I could concentrate, and how to prop up my struggling immune system or calm it down when I needed it the most. I was able to start reading what my body needed and then deliver it. A skill that I use *every single day* of my life. There are no days off.

The people I know who are the happiest and have the best quality of life pay attention to their food, and I do not mean calorie counting or cutting whole food groups because of some fad seen on Instagram. I mean tuning into what works for the individual and then being flexible within that. After all, the fact is that, as humans, everything we consume has an effect on us. Not all of us react the same, nor does every reaction equal pain. Some things help us feel more energized and capable.

Neither am I saying that all the fun foods, like chocolate, have to go away (I think that almond-milk gluten-free chocolate should be its own food group!); it is truly unique for each person. But when those people spent even just a couple of weeks looking into what they put in their bodies, they found patterns of emotional, physical, and mental responses, and using that data, they were then better prepared to get the most out of their bodies by feeding them what actually worked for them. I don't believe in cutting out whole food groups just because it's fashionable to do so, but I definitely think it's worth working out what's going to help you. For some of us, this process may be motivated by a fear of getting sick or prompted by curiosity or a health concern, but eventually it transforms and becomes a case of "I feel awesome when I do this, and I live a really full life now, so why wouldn't I do it?" This is not about taking things away, this is actually about giving yourself more options that help you.

These lessons made me think about why the concept of a boundary versus a restriction made such a difference to me. I started to wonder if it was the same for every one of us. And what I have observed is that humans do not do well when they are restricted, but we thrive when we know our boundaries. So much of human history, from my point of view, shows repeated patterns of societal restriction (of varying kinds) where our resulting behaviour and wellbeing is poor. That is, until we find ways to change the restriction into a boundary. When we change it to a boundary, we demonstrate patterns of evolution. They happen so seamlessly it's almost impossible to recognise the difference between the phases, but in action the difference is stark. I encourage you to notice it them within your own life. Restriction tends to bring out the worst in us. It certainly did in me. Our nature is to rebel and revolt against it. We become destructive to ourselves as well as to others. We speak out of turn, we brim with anger and frustration, we give off toxic draining energy, we binge eat boxes of doughnuts, we give up on our most precious dreams, we pick fights with those we care about, we become less capable in our jobs and unhealthier in every possible way, and we can become quite depressed, anxious, and despondent.

However, when we turn our restrictions into useful boundaries, we flourish. The best of us comes to the forefront. We become more open to others, more empathetic, healthier, happier, more creative, and more confident to boot. We get better at our jobs and businesses, we become better leaders and parents, and we embrace more of what the world has to offer. We actually make the most of the time we are given. This is because boundaries provide options and choices and help us negotiate a way to get what we want from life and often from our bodies.

Food may or may not be your box of restriction, but I'd bet my bottom dollar that you have had or do have one in your life. And you probably didn't enjoy having to face it either. You likely dug your heels in with stubborn frustration and became a little unpleasant to be around. Restriction steals away choice and options and suffocates hope in the process.

When we are in a box of restriction, it is unpleasant and sometimes feels like there is little we can do about it. But in my experience, that's just not the case most of the time. So next time you find yourself restricted, take a big breath, and start feeling for the ceiling, the walls, the edges, and the spots that have a little give. They are there. When you find them, push. Push and change that box from a restriction into a boundary, a box with the flexibility to mold to what you want and need.

This is a skill that takes time to develop but is really the cornerstone of how we, as a species, have survived on this planet for so long. When we are restricted, we don't just become complacent, shrug our shoulders and die. No, we rise within and bend the restriction into a boundary that works for us. We get the creative part of our brains flowing. We let the lizard brain have a sleep-in and start operating from within our more evolved self. We research our options. We pay attention. We learn, and we thrive.

The lessons I have learned from learning to operate within a boundary instead of a restriction have been incredibly transferrable. In business meetings these days, I will often say to a potential partner that I want to know where my boundaries are because then I will know how much room I have to play with. I think this is true in every area of life. Because everything is connected. So next time you find the walls closing in, give freedom, choice, and hope back to yourself by pushing until that box bends to your will!

WELLNESS TIP:
Mindful-Living Tracker

Track your life. What you are doing and consuming and how you react to things can go on your tracker each day. At the end of two or three weeks, patterns will begin to emerge, and you will be able to adjust your quality of life by removing the things that do not serve you and adding in things that may. Below is an example of what a tracker might look like and what kind of information you could put in it.

Time & Day	Activity/Food	Emotional Response	Physical Response	Mental Response
Monday morning	30 minutes of running. Cereal with milk, cup of coffee, glass of water, sliced apple.	Felt calm after the run.	Felt good after the run, but really dehydrated before I even started. Got really hungry before lunch. Stomach got very growly. Lips and mouth feel very dry.	Felt very awake after the run, but when my stomach grew growly, I started to become agitated and couldn't concentrate.

Time & Day	Activity/Food	Emotional Response	Physical Response	Mental Response
Monday lunch	Chicken-salad sandwich and a coffee. Ate it while working at my desk.	Feeling a bit sensitive and agitated.	Very sore in my legs and glutes, but I also have a headache, and I feel very tired now too. Did a poop; wasn't very solid. Bloated and cramping.	Finding it difficult to get things done. Keep getting distracted, and I am also getting angry at my body for being tired.
Monday night	Pasta with Napoli sauce, glass of wine, glass of water.

Watched TV, went on Instagram. | A bit angry or easily annoyed and grumpy. | Very fatigued and stiff, sluggish. I feel uncomfortably full.

Breakouts on my nose. Skin is dry. | My mind is very wired even though my body is tired. Finding it hard to stop my mind chatter so I can get to sleep. |

8

DON'T WAIT FOR PERMISSION

Underdog is another label I have felt a personal affinity with for most of my life. Partially because of falling into the invisible illness category, but also because I am small-statured and female. Even in a pair of stilettos, with the biggest of power stances and wearing a blazer, I am not even close to head height with the average person. And, as a general rule, I haven't warranted too much attention. To say I have been overlooked and underestimated isn't speculation on my part, it's just a fact (at least from my view down here).

I've had some fairly good motivation in my life, though, to fight for what I want and need. Having a disease that can stop me from even being able to leave the house means I am fully aware of how much experience I could miss out on. And spending a fair chunk of my life sicker than most, I have also become painfully aware of how fragile and fleeting this thing called life actually is. It's so incredibly easy for time to pass me by when I am under the weather. It's simply too convenient for obstacles to steal my future.

One of the advantages that has come with my lived human experience has been that I have been in both the driver's seat and the passenger's seat at differing times. I know that the longer one avoids taking chances on themselves, the easier it gets to justify merely existing.

What I have observed is that, for many people, it becomes so simple to work under the assumption that there's "plenty of time" to make things happen. And this kind of thinking is easy to reinforce by not taking action on opportunities, dreams, risks, and hope. It used to drive me up the wall, watching all these healthy people just let life happen to them when they had the option to do so much more with it. I had to fight to get out of bed or the bathroom half the time, while they were complaining about their lives yet were unwilling to change them even though they could. These days, I recognize that not everyone wants to change their lives; some people are genuinely satisfied with things as they are. Kudos to them and to you if you're one of them. However, I have to say, I haven't met too many genuinely satisfied people.

I can make months' worth of plans and schedule my days with dozens of fabulous things, but the truth is that I will probably have to reschedule and shuffle things around a bit more than the average person. While it happens less and less often because I live through wellness, from time to time my disease can see me go from fully functional one day to bedridden or hospitalized very quickly. Living under that kind of umbrella of unpredictability has led me to believe that everything we face as humans is quite temporary by its very nature. That used to make me quite sad, but not anymore. This fleeting fragility is what makes life so special, such a privilege, such a beautiful blessing, even the crappy bits. None of us know when things will change, really. It will suddenly go away one day. That's just how it is. But this is not a reason to be forlorn at all. It's a reason to get out into the world and own yourself, your influence and your power. YASSSS people. Self-Validation is where it is at!

If you've ever come across someone who just seems to sail through life, with job promotions and other opportunities falling into their laps, please know that is not a reflection of who I am at all. Nothing has ever happened for me that way. Ever. Nope. Everything that has come into my life (aside from the obvious), both good and bad, is because of me.

I am the common denominator in my own equation. Funnily enough, you are in yours too.

Early on in my adult life, I had a string of near misses. I'd start jobs, working hard and diligently, all while trying to please everyone and earn my stripes in whatever field I was in. And I would end up being completely disregarded for roles or underestimated in my capabilities. I was continuously told I was "not ready" for things I had worked long and hard for. I would be told I didn't have enough experience to do something I knew I could do. "Too nice," "too eager," "too young," and "too unwell," also followed me around. I was always just "too" much of something. Very often, these claims would be made by people quite literally sizing me up with their eyes. I knew that much of what was being said was just a politically correct way of telling me to stop trying because I was a small female who took time off work because I was sick and had opinions people didn't want to hear.

I know there have been times I didn't get a job because whatever company I was working for had never hired a woman for that role. Sometimes it was because my opinion was mistaken for having *emotion*. (Human beings need to express emotion; it is healthy and what we are designed to do. Read that again.) Sometimes my disease was considered a significant weakness. I don't resent any of it. It taught me a lot.

After a lot of soul-searching and stressing, I came to the conclusion that it didn't matter what I did to adjust myself to be less of something instead of too much of something, like changing my clothes, the tone of my voice, how fast or slow I worked, and so on. I could not change the three fundamental things that seemed to be my obstacles. I was always going to be a short female with a chronic disease. For a while, I was incredibly frustrated by this fact. Did I play the "it's not fair" game with myself sometimes? Yes, indeed, I did, and I was great at it! But I also worked out that playing that game just made me feel worse and certainly wasn't a way to find solutions.

Because I had spent so long mastering the art of resilience fortified by facing continuous pain and uncertainty, I knew what I was capable of. That confidence and desire to take on the world was something I earned, but seemed to be deeply threatening to others when I used it in the workplace. I was eager to be of service, and when I turned my mind to a task, I would deliver not just a satisfactory outcome but a great one. Not because I wanted the glory, but because I expected myself to deliver high quality with anything I did. A job I did was never a job half done—something I learned from my amazing father. I knew that, if I had to, I could take on most people's roles, and with some serious devotion and willingness to fall flat on my face, I would eventually be able to do it. I knew that because there were so many days when even getting out of bed could have stopped me, yet it didn't. This doesn't mean I was better at a job than anyone else, but I believe humans are capable of so much with the right motivation and thinking, and I applied that to myself.

I saw my resilience and work ethic as pros, not cons, but quite often other people didn't agree with me on that. Their world was black and white, and I lived in the grey. They saw a lack of experience on paper as a sign I couldn't do something. They saw my illness as a reason not to give me a shot at something more. I had become so used to having to live chunks of life between bouts of illness that I had become adept at getting things done efficiently and spotting problems before they happened. A career on stage will also teach you a lot about having to "get on with the show." So when a task was thrown at me, I didn't approach it with a nonchalant attitude of "I will get it done later." For me, it was "I am doing it now, and while I am here, were you aware that no process for this part of the task exists and that's going to cost us all time and money?" Turns out, lots of managers don't love people like this on their teams. I do.

I was never, ever rude or mean or condescending, and I was abundantly aware that I didn't know everything and that I would not always be right. But the things I had conviction in and had the stats or facts on I owned. Staff of the same authority level as me tended to like me. I would come into a workplace, and within a week, could understand what they were frustrated about after being there for years. I gave voice to their gripes, but I also ensured that I provided solutions. Management just wanted me to go away, although my male counterparts and "well" people doing the same thing were accepted. And when I had bent over backward to try to make things work but failed to do so, I would leave, recognizing that I was never going to be allowed to move forward if I stayed. Because life could already be hard for me day to day, I sure as hell wasn't prepared to live what time I had at 50 percent of my capacity or having someone else cap my experiences.

My biggest issue was that I was waiting. Waiting for permission to do what I was good at. Waiting for a sign that it was time to let my full, authentic personality out. Waiting for the right opportunity to present itself, or for the right person to recognize what I could do and actually help me rise. Waiting for someone to ignore their own attitude to my disease, and instead, recognise my human potential. Waiting, waiting, waiting. And as I waited, my precious time was slipping away from me. It's not that I was in a hurry at all. I was not frantic or panicked. I just wanted to fill my life with experiences. I wanted to leave the planet with stories, knowing I had given everything a go. I wanted to know what I was good at and what was not in my wheelhouse. I wanted the good, the bad, and the ugly. Hell, I was living with some of the bad and ugly already—I wanted to taste the good. I wanted to demonstrate to myself and others like me that it could be done. I wanted to do things that I desired because I could, not despite or in spite of something else. And I was gaining plenty of experience with the word *no*. So clearly it was going to have to be me that got me where I wanted to go.

When I made the transition from dance teacher to choreographer, I really wanted to work on the television and film side of the industry, but I found that the limited number of jobs available in Australia were going to the same handful of choreographers, repetitively. In fact, most of the time, producers would call choreographers they had worked with directly to book them for upcoming projects. Breaking your way into that part of the industry was tricky and hard to navigate. On the rare occasion that there was an open call for choreographers, I would attend and be told that, while my body of work was good and I was capable of doing fusion (for example, mixing Balinese dance with hip-hop, or contemporary with Latin) which gave me a unique edge, I wasn't experienced enough on film sets. But how do you get experience when no one gives it to you? My answer was to go ahead and make opportunities for myself.

So, in collaboration with a local music group, I put together a music video and ran the production myself. This meant I had my hands across advertising; auditioning; working with the costume, hair, and makeup artists that we had hired; location set up; and scheduling everyone, from the camera team to the extras being shot in the film. And of course I was creating the actual dancing and overall vision for the music video. I was on the phone convincing people to get involved in this unknown project and largely calling on my own faith and my stage experience to make it work. Doing this so hands-on, I was building relationships with all the different members of the team because it was important to me that they each had their signature across the project. I wanted whatever I did to help them, too, so they could proudly use this work as part of their portfolios and help them get more jobs in the industry.

Applying all the things I knew from the stage and from doing musicals, I decided that it would be best to break down the choreography into shorter sections, with music cut to the lengths of those phrases of dance. This way, the editor could more effectively place the pieces back together without having to look for a spot in a flowing dance movement to do a cut. It's easy to lose timing in a flowing piece of art on screen because we are talking hundredths of a second, and nothing annoys me more than badly timed dancing on screen. Ugh! I also knew this would sustain the dancers and make it easier for lighting changes. It meant I could schedule us to film in sections, and that way, I was not asking dancers to do overly athletic sections for days on end. I didn't want anyone to walk off that set thinking I had burned them out. All of these little things that I used as my style of choreography and management were about care and efficiency and wellness. I was told later that it made a real impact on the set. From completing that project, I had a music video to my name. I had gained a lot of experience and learning in all areas of the production from being so hands-on and collaborative, and I gained a huge circle of like-minded creative folks to work with.

As I moved through the industry, that music video helped me get other music videos, and film projects too. It served its purpose from that point of view, but I gained so much more than that. I was able to call on this fantastic group of artists for other projects as I was offered roles in them. I was able to recommend them for jobs, sometimes even give them to them myself as I gained a little more power as a player in the scene. They would call on me to do work when someone asked them for a recommendation too. I was able to show my fusion skills on film because I wasn't answering to anyone but me, and that led to me being able to put fusion dance on stages and on screen and even to teach it to up-and-coming professionals. And by doing more projects my way, I was also able to reduce the hours that I needed to be very physical to the minimum, making it easier for me to manage my health at the same time.

None of this was going to come to me by waiting for it to happen. I hustled and ended up with so much more than I had expected from the process. That hustle got me into rooms with other artists and directors that would never have been open to me. I was offered projects that never would have come my way. I had people reaching out to me in fashion, dramatic film, private events like birthday parties, community and government events, and interstate projects as a result of taking this step.

Later on, in a role outside the dance industry, I was hired by a company to improve morale, end the high turnover rate in a creative team, and enhance the delivery timelines of the service they offered to their client base. I knew I was capable of doing the role, as everything they had described I had mastered in the dance industry. Being a choreographer ends up meaning you do a bit of everything, so everything I learned there applied to "real world" office jobs. However, the management team at the company wasn't so sure because of how I looked on paper. They offered me a junior version of the role I had interviewed for instead of the lead title, but with the same responsibility and hours. I justified in my head that I just had to prove myself through doing good work, and then the official title (and pay) would be mine. I took the junior role and diligently set to work on the tasks I had been given, hoping to get the promotion.

In less than six months, I had delivered everything they had asked of me and more. My team ran like clockwork. I had improved morale by introducing "cup of tea" time each week where I gave the team a chance to vent, bond, and plan for the week ahead. I learned about my team, what kind of things made them tick, and rerouted work from just ending up in anyone's lap to ending up in the lap of the person who wanted that challenge the most. The staff turnover came to a grinding halt. We were getting better work to the clients in a timelier fashion, and along the way, I had set up processes that helped streamline the way other departments communicated. I had nailed it.

One day, I was sitting at my desk when I was asked by the branch manager to sit in on an interview with a new staff member. As the interview started, I realized that the company was seeking someone to do the senior version of my role. I was gutted. I hadn't even been asked by the management team. I had been entirely dismissed. So after the interview, I expressed my disappointment and highlighted that I was already doing the job, that I had achieved even more than they had asked, and that what I had done was improving their bottom line. I wanted to know why I had been disregarded for the role. I was told that I had done everything right, but that other staff who had been at the company longer still hadn't been promoted, so it would upset the apple cart too much if I was promoted into the role, being so new. I was also told that some clients would likely not take me seriously because I "looked too young" and that some clients were a bit "old school" and I would "not be what they expected" and that they couldn't put someone in that role who might need "time off due to being sick." In other words, I was too small, too diseased, and too feminine to do the role.

Even though I had been doing the role already, I had taken no more time off than anyone else, and for a bargain pay rate, I might add! But I had told them I had Crohn's because I was trying not to be invisible for once. I was outraged and so disappointed that my obstacles were in my way again. This situation was something I just couldn't get past, and I knew if I stayed, I would be showing up at work every day seething. That kind of toxicity would actually set me into a Crohn's flare-up, or at minimum, increase the pain levels in my body, making my days that much harder to get through.

I had two options: stay and get sick or hustle my way into something better. I started making phone calls to friends and colleagues to see if an opportunity was out there for me. I reached out to the people on social media I was inspired by most to see if they would respond. I told my network of pals that I was jumping ship, which meant they were at the ready to be references for me as needed.

Low and behold, one of the people I had looked up to online was prepared to meet me. I jumped at the chance to meet, and when I did, I threw my résumé right out the window. It was time to start selling me and stop relying on what other people would derive from my experience on paper. I presented my stats and told him what I could do for him. I told him what I lacked and what my strengths were. I told him how my experiences in dance and business could be easily transferred. And I got the job! It took me less than two weeks to make the move. And the move I made put me in a role that utilized all my skills. I was paid accordingly and now had access to rooms full of people that I never would have been able to meet before. All the people I admired in business associated with the company I worked for. Getting that role also meant I was able to build relationships with the people who were making power moves around the world. Watching how these people operated was the biggest form of education in so many areas of business.

I was expanding my skills and learning how to be confident in my abilities and own them. I learned how to move and work even faster in this environment. I got used to people talking about money in millions instead of thousands. And from this role, I grew a network of people that helped me in business myself. These amazing people helped me to grow more confident in myself as a leader. They didn't think of my being little or female or having a disease as an issue.

Would I have ever got there had I waited my turn to take a larger role at the previous job? No. I might still be there being undervalued. I didn't wait. I hustled.

Right before I launched my own business, Corethentic, I worked in the fitness industry for a time. I had earned my qualifications as a personal trainer and group fitness instructor because I wanted to know more about the human body. I also felt that I had worked out a system that could be sold to the fitness industry even though it called on a lot of my dance experience. So once I had my certifications, I made a strategic decision to work in gyms and studios so that I could better understand the inner workings of the industry and see where my idea might fit. I specifically took on roles that allowed me to get an education in the entire business model. I sold gym memberships, chased up clients in debt, had personal training clients, and ran group fitness and small group fitness classes in many styles. I made up classes for gyms to use, managed the gym floor (Please put your weights away when you finish with them. Love, from anyone who's ever worked in a gym) and worked with gym managers to track their numbers. It was like getting a fitness business degree!

When I would work with my PT clients, from my time in dance I had an extra bag of skills to pull from, and I didn't hesitate to have my clients use them if it was appropriate for their needs. My clients thrived. Their health concerns didn't pose as obstacles to me, as I lived in a body that needed a little more specialized care myself. The other trainers in the gyms would stare at me from across the floor as I demonstrated movements, used equipment in nontraditional ways, and brought my flavor to the gym scene. I was certainly different, and of course I was still the short, "little" girl. I wasn't huge and bulky, and often the trainers would be surprised by how strong I was or the ways I could use my body. I didn't look like a personal trainer. I wasn't deterred by seeming like a fish out of water in the gym environment. I was a fish out of water no matter where I was. I was tapping into what was authentic for my clients and me, and it worked.

Some of the other trainers would watch me through the windows when I ran gym classes. They would often tell me after a class that they'd never thought of "doing a move like that" and that they wanted to use it themselves. Slowly, my skills in wellness, even some of the breathing techniques I was teaching my clients, started to be used by others around the gym. It wasn't that odd after a few months. Still different, but not odd. And I saw wellness slowly be normalized in the gym environment, even though that term hadn't reached the mainstream yet. My client numbers were up, and attendance in my classes was solid and regular. I was using all of this feedback to confirm what I already knew: the system I had designed to keep me flourishing was working on other people. The gym managers were sending me all the "hard clients" with spinal injuries, arthritis, nerve issues, chronic fatigue, and more, and these clients loved what I was delivering. They felt welcome and safe in the gym for the first time. I was thrilled to be of service. It's everything I had wanted to achieve with my formula.

I figured that the gyms I was working with might be interested in launching my system as a test. Since I was doing good work, and because they kept using me as the example of a good trainer to others with the same job, I expected that I would at least be given the opportunity to have a conversation or to pitch them my ideas.

When I asked, I was told immediately and in no uncertain terms, "NO." I kept trying, often with a different pitch, to try to sell it. I kept being told no. They were not even willing to have a discussion about it. When I pushed harder, I was advised that "there is no market for what you do, Flic. It just won't work." I was told that my business couldn't work because I "couldn't possibly be the face of a business in fitness with a disease." I countered that I was being sent all the clients that were considered hard work and that they were going from being casual clients to people who came into the gym several times per week because they thought of me as living proof that one could still have a quality of life with a disease. I knew those clients would come to classes if they were made available, and I also knew that we could corner the aged care and female fitness markets with what I was offering. I asked if I could try doing classes in off-peak times and again was told no.

I was dumbfounded. I had the market, the numbers, and the proof that it worked, but I was still being told no. I wasn't even being given a shot. I was so deflated. I had waited and tried to earn my stripes and was denied permission. Again.

So I decided to be a CEO from then on. I gave myself the promotion and got on with it. I put that hat on and started hustling. I waved goodbye to the gyms and took on a temporary office role to earn some regular bucks while I worked on my business formula and got all my ducks lined up in a row. It didn't take me long to be ready to launch. I bypassed the gyms entirely and started to make calls to all the dance studios I had worked with, trying to find a proper venue at a rate I could afford to pay. I got online and started reaching out to everyone I didn't yet know in the fitness industry, just so that I could build relationships and keep learning. I was convinced that what I had would also work online, and I wanted to understand the potential of that space, too, because so many of us with chronic illness can't get to a gym or studio to train regularly. So I set up meetings with people all over the world so I could educate myself.

Through those calls, I was able to learn from and connect with the people who really made the industry tick. I was able to be of service to them in a multitude of ways (business should always be a two-way street). And from these calls, I was being put in rooms with people who noticed potential in what I did. I was getting media coverage by selecting the events to show up at and speak or demonstrate at that made the most sense for my goals.

I sought out and hired my first staff, legendary human beings that are blessings in my life, who helped to craft and give a face other than my own to what I was doing. We jumped into the virtual fitness space and the offline-class space with a burst.

But none of what I have achieved was done alone or by chance. I would not have been in those rooms or had an online platform without having hustled to get there. People opened doors for me that made it possible, but I had to bust the first doors open myself. I had a lot of doors closed in my face along the way. A lot of people just wouldn't talk to me. I was an unknown in the scene, and I was talking about wellness before it was mainstream. I was also talking about chronic pain and invisible illness and aged care and women's health, and none of that seemed sexy, but I knew there was a gap in the market there because I fit in the gap myself!

I have now had the opportunity to keynote at big events that never would have touched me with a ten-foot pole before. I have been interviewed and recorded and filmed by people in many industries and have had my work mentioned in magazines like *Women's Health Australia* and published by big brands like Lorna Jane. Most importantly, I have had the opportunity to sit down with people just like me who have spent years suffering in silence and feeling hopeless and have had them literally cry with relief because, through what I have put together, they feel seen and heard for the first time in their lives. They feel like there is hope. And that's what I wanted to do in the first place: give hope, an alternative, and be an example.

I am not special at all. I am not describing anything fancy. I built a business. I am not a Fortune 500 mogul (watch this space). But I faced obstacles to get there. I faced them head-on by opting not to wait for the right time or for someone's permission. I hustled instead, and I made it happen. I see so clearly how my path to wellness translated to how I navigated my way here. I hustled to wellness too. I wasn't going to get permission from the medical industry to live as I do. I made the decision, I did the work, I asked the questions and made it happen. **Wellness gave me my humanness. My humanness amplified my inner hustler.**

We all have reasons not to do things. I bet you have plenty of obstacles too, perhaps way more than me. But nothing changes until *you* do. And your time on this planet is mighty precious and is not unlimited. Your obstacles are just as fleeting, and your life is just as fragile as everyone else's. Whatever it is you face doesn't define you. What you do with the time you have does. So stop waiting for permission to live the quality of life you desire, and start hustling your way there, in your own unique way.

WELLNESS TIP:
Hydrate

Water is required for your body to do pretty much anything you can think of, including think!

If you struggle to get an adequate amount in each day, slowly introduce it to your system over a period of weeks so you don't feel bloated. Wake up and drink half a glass of water before you do anything else. This helps flush out the toxins your body has accumulated overnight in its natural detoxing process. Stimulants like coffee can dehydrate the body. If this is the first thing you consume in the day, you may be placing extra pressure on your body because it will be unable to properly release its toxins. Each week increase your water intake in the morning by another half a glass. Once you are used to doing this, your body will be less inclined to rebel when you drink it during the day, making it much easier to increase your intake in general. Oh and by the way, you will pee a lot for a few weeks. This is good, not bad. It means your body will finally get the chance to flush out all the toxins that are likely making you feel more sluggish than you currently realize. Eventually it calms down.

Your mental, emotional, and physical self will love you for it. In fact, no matter what time of day it is, go grab a glass and take a drink right now!

9

WORK SMART

The majority of the people I have met throughout my years have been raised or educated to equate working hard with success and even with their personal identity and sense of self-worth. For most of my life, I subscribed to that model of thinking, and the behavior that stems from it too. I was so good at sticking to the formula that I left next to no time for play.

My head was filled with all the slogans that had been drummed into me: "You have to work hard if you want to get anywhere in life." "Work now. Play later." "Working hard is a sacrifice, but it's worth it." They ran on repeat like a tape in my head. I also believed that anything outside of work was some kind of reward that I had to earn through . . . (drumroll please) working hard.

The base idea is OK, really. Things in life do not come for free, and it is certainly important to understand that working gives you money and that you need money to pay for food. However, the issue is that when we look at life as work and reward or work and play, we are trying to make our journeys black and white. None of us live in black and white. Our journeys are filled with grey. So by segmenting life into just two distinct buckets and balancing our sense of worth or our ability to be a success against them, we are setting ourselves up to fall. When you have only two buckets and society has deemed the first one, work, as the only real importance, everything else gets dumped into the play bucket even if it doesn't belong there. That often means that our health also finds itself in the wrong bucket.

I used to justify the way I approached my work by saying, "But I love what I do," even though I never made room for this elusive "play" that had been dangled in front of me like a carrot. And truthfully, I did love what I did and still do, but it is not and never should have been all there was. Yet because of my thinking, I sacrificed spending time with friends and going to special milestone events and put literally everything that wasn't work to the side. That's an entirely unrealistic way to live, yet so many of us do it. Where's all the grey gone?

The issue with work is that, technically speaking, it's never really done. There is always more to do. Even when you are working on one task, your brain is learning and thinking of better ways to do it, other approaches to take, thinking of all the other things associated with your current task that now also need to be done to support this task's completion, and more. It's a trap to think that if you work hard, you will earn your playtime. It is a tragedy that so many of us operate on this mentality of working endlessly for rewards we never allow ourselves the time or space to have because we are too busy working for them. No matter what you do, if you have this way of thinking, there will always be some other magical hoop that appears that you think you have to jump through before you can relax.

But I do not subscribe to that thinking anymore. Saying I have changed the tune that dictated most of my life would be an understatement, and while I am no master at "playing," I am much better than ever before, and I am so thankful that's the case. My health is in its own special bucket now! I no longer work hard for anything; I now work smart, and there is a huge difference between the two. Let me explain.

When my husband and I made our way over to Silicon Valley (San Francisco, USA) to be part of the startup scene, it meant uprooting our entire lives and waving goodbye to everyone we had ever known or loved, in order to seize the day. We had an opportunity to take a leap of faith and get some life experience that not everyone is fortunate enough to get. We wanted to see how the biggest, most innovative, and influential businesses in the world operated, and so when we made the decision to move countries, we went all-in to make it happen.

For me, this meant drawing a line in the sand and ending my professional dance career. It also meant I now had more than two decades' worth of vast experience to try to apply to industries and roles I had never been in before. But I had worked hard my entire life and was convinced that what I would experience in the Valley wouldn't test me that much. Paying my bills by being a dancer in Australia was *tough*, so the Valley didn't worry me much. Boy, oh boy, was I naïve!

Silicon Valley blew my mind, and I worked out very quickly that, in order to succeed there, I was going to have to do a lot of growing—fast. Culturally, there were big differences in the approach to business and life, and how we communicated too. Australians are down-to-earth, laid back, and like to enjoy life. We are also pretty humble and tend to downplay our strengths and success and only talk about them if someone else has brought them up as a topic of conversation. Conversely, Americans seemed to be super confident, loud, and unafraid of other people's perceptions of them. They literally yelled at each other from across the street, which was classed as a "conversation" (something I never quite got used to). Americans put their strengths and success into their opening introductions when they said hello. They were always "on," always looking for opportunity, and everyone was in the Valley to win big. Being around them initially was very intimidating to me. So the first thing I had to do was get comfortable with what Aussies would call "talking yourself up"—telling people what I was good at and why I was worth talking to, a skill that has been helpful but was not natural to me.

When I entered the workforce there, I was overwhelmed. Not only was everyone's personality big, but there was a lot of competition between people who had a very different approach to business. There were some unique advantages to their cultural approach to entrepreneurship. It was surprisingly easy to get a coffee meeting with a major CEO just to chat; whereas in Australia, you had to work your way through a long network of people before you were able to even ask a CEO if they'd be willing to talk to you. I loved that change but didn't like many of the others, like work environments changing minute to minute, loads of competitive politics between in-house teams, and high turnover rates of staff. It made getting to know people on a deeper level very challenging. I felt like a real alien. I recall sitting on the edge of my bed in the first week of Valley life balling my eyes out because I couldn't understand how I would ever be able to survive in such a competitive, fast-paced, and cutthroat environment.

I knew the Valley was filled with exceptionally talented and successful people. It's why I went there—to learn from the best. But even though I saw success unfold in front of my eyes, I didn't see any joyous reactions to success. I recall sitting on a train heading to work, and on board, like every other day, people were wearing T-shirts with their company logos. *There are so many of them; it looks like everyone is going to a sports carnival wearing their team colors*, I thought. A group of people in matching shirts climbed aboard, and people started clapping and congratulating them on a successful IPO (initial public offering: when a company becomes a publicly traded entity). But the team that had just done the IPO looked devastated, exhausted, gaunt, and very unhappy. There were no smiles, and they seemed barely able to acknowledge the congratulations they were receiving. Within seconds, they all had their laptops out, like the rest of us, and worked the whole journey to their stop. I was baffled. These people had reached the apex of Valley success, and it looked like someone had just passed away. This is how success so often presented itself while I was there.

Even parties were not relaxing events used to unwind. Everyone was still networking, talking about business, or competing with each other through beer pong, or while a party raged, a room of developers would still be madly coding away. One group of people would be panicking that they didn't have the money to make payroll that week, and another would be talking about having just gotten a ten-million-dollar investment. If they hadn't opened their mouths and explained their situation, you might not have been able to tell them apart. Success and failure seemed to foster the same results.

The hours of work were completely unrealistic. Sure, a company might be open from eight a.m. to five p.m., but that didn't mean those were the hours its employees worked. Often people were in well before opening time and for hours after closing time. Weekends just meant working from home, and holidays still meant checking email, jumping on video calls, and generally being available. One might do ten to twelve hours in the office, then go home and do another two to four hours. Silicon Valley seemed to work on a nonstop basis.

All of the huge companies had perks, like in-house catering, snacks, work drinks, and social activities. I've never seen such consumption of pizza, beer, Red Bull, and coffee in my entire life. Hackathons, where engineers, developers, and more gather for full weekends to create or innovate new products or code, fueled largely by pizza and Red Bull, were common.

Very quickly, life meant socialising and working with the same people all the time and doing, talking about, or thinking about work around the clock.

Watching the behavior of everyone around me, the message was pretty clear. You were expected to work hard and show no sign that this amount of work affected you negatively at all. I had observed people being "blacklisted" for admitting that they were struggling, and immediately knew that if I talked about my own issues, I would be creating another obstacle to my success in this environment. It was hard enough having to rephrase my sentences and adjust my tone of voice in order to be understood with my accent! People weighed your value and potential for success against the number of hours you were willing to put in. And despite all the opportunities for achievement, all the advantages of being able to work with the most amazing people in the world, or having the best résumé as a result of scoring a job at one of the "unicorns" (rare, super-successful startups like Facebook, Uber, etc.), I really didn't meet many people who seemed satisfied or, even rarer, those who seemed healthy. Mostly, I would hear people say, "I am so exhausted, but I just have to keep going."

Mental, physical, and emotional health issues surrounded me in the people I met who'd worked tirelessly to succeed. Many of them moved on because the pace wasn't sustainable for them. A lot of them got sick. Some of them seemed to lose their personal identity in the process. The term *burnout* wasn't in circulation back then like it is now, but that is what I was witnessing—people burning out in every possible way around me. In the wake of business success or failure, I saw people looking broken and unwell and having to rebuild themselves. The successes and failures seemed to take an equal toll on the founders of businesses and the staff that helped carry the company over the goal line.

Little priority and importance were placed on mental, emotional, or physical health. Not once did I hear any company talk about this while I was there. I had such a hard time accepting that business success could mean so much personal unhappiness or ill health. I wanted to be well, happy, and successful. Surely that had to be possible!

Like everyone else, I was in the Valley to learn, grow, succeed, and prove myself. And despite my knowledge of health, I fell into the trap of "working hard," too, because I mirrored my environment, which was a BIG lesson. It was all I saw and heard about, and therefore, all I absorbed. Very quickly, I was working the same hours, worried about the same kinds of stresses, and weighing myself against "working hard" to gather how valuable or capable I was. I was taking the calls on weekends and working into the wee hours of the morning. I wasn't taking care of my body, and I certainly wasn't doing anything for my mind, except reading business books in order to be as successful as my counterparts. I wanted to be the best in business, so I copied what I saw, which was a total dedication to working hard.

I sustained this seven-days-a-week-style work pace for three years before life seemed to have lost all color, and I felt like I had pulled everything I could from the experience of being in the Valley. I'd had the opportunity to meet some of my idols and even work for them. I had worked for a few people that deeply disappointed me. Not everyone in life is who they seem to be. But the ones who impressed me were Gary Vaynerchuck, Lesley Gold, and Marc Alexander, who gave me a huge business education without knowing it. Under their wings, I had learned how to pitch and sell, pivot quickly, prepare investment decks, speak to boards of directors, understand loads of investment jargon, and apply my entertainment skills to sectors like PR, social media, and IoT. I got to see behind the curtain and learn from innovators and disruptors who have fundamentally changed how we function across the globe. I learned that my skills were assets instead of cons, which made me confident I could play in the big leagues in a C-level role. I learned to manage teams and developed better leadership skills. I have made friends with people I deeply admire and respect, who helped me blend my Aussie thinking with American thinking to get a nice mixture of both; I am now an Aussie-can. It was the ultimate business degree on steroids, and I am forever changed and grateful for going through it.

On the flip side of that coin, I learned more about what *not* to do from my time in the Valley than what *to* do. I returned to Australia entirely burned out. I hit rock bottom hard and fast. My body and mind fell apart the second my feet were safely back on Australian soil. I had worked myself so hard that I had adrenal fatigue. My body was firing off chemicals at weird times as a result, so I would lie awake for nights on end, entirely unable to sleep for even a minute, covered in sweat. I was emotionally all over the place, crying and angry and deeply lost. I was continuously sick with every bug that came my way because my poor immune system couldn't operate, and my Crohn's and IBS were flogging me daily. It made it hard to keep any kind of job, let alone start my business. I was a mess. Working hard practically broke me. It took a monumental amount of effort to overcome burnout and rebuild myself.

While I was in the process of putting the pieces back together, I couldn't shake the idea that there had to be a way to achieve success without becoming burned out. I could not reconcile the idea of putting myself through that stress again for my own business. If I was going to do it, it had to be sustainable for me. I decided my life was way too precious to spend it flogging myself and then being unhappy even if I managed to achieve something. So I started to research burnout and the things that help people thrive. Also, I knew upfront I could not structure my business in the same way as most people. A seven-days-a-week lifestyle was unrealistic for me. I had to work out how to be successful but operate like I was already semiretired. I had to bring myself into the equation and avoid mirroring those around me.

I was not surprised to see that burnout is a huge issue and that it's affecting people all over the world, not just in business but also in other careers, study, and home life. In fact, it's having a significant impact on physical and mental health. There is even research drawing links between burnout and suicide. I understood firsthand the physiological manifestations of stress on the mind and body because I was living it. I was disturbed to find once I looked closer that this was not a Valley issue, but instead an everywhere issue. I had just seen it for the first time in the Valley due to the intensity of it there.

I then studied to become a wellness coach and gained a diploma in neuroplasticity so that I could get a greater grasp on the mental loops that prevent so many of us from breaking the behavioral patterns that lead to us being unwell or dissatisfied and burned out. I knew that there was a lot of psychology weaved into the way we dismiss the needs of our bodies to satisfy our need to fit in with our peers. I wanted to learn how to redirect my thinking so that one day I could help others do it themselves.

I absorbed as much as I could about what we are as humans, mammals, and primates. I learned that we build communities everywhere we go instinctually. Our workplaces, businesses, gyms, social groups, friends, supermarkets, favorite cafés, and families are just some of these.

They not only provide food, water, and shelter, but they also allow us to feel safe, seen, heard, and valued. These things are what I would call the drivers of how we function. In fact, when we find ourselves in communities that do not promote or provide the opportunity to have our fundamental needs met, we cannot sustain. It affects our health in all ways. All aspects of our well-being need to be supported in our environment for our bodies and minds to function well.

When I combined my experience and understanding of the body and mind with what I had observed in the Valley, I recognized immediately what was missing and what had been bugging me all along. The biggest issue was that we had forgotten that we are humans.

Humans have a brain that is aware that it is a brain. Use your brain to think about that for a second. We are "Inceptioning" ourselves all the time. We have links between the mind, body, and emotion, which operate as a two-way street. Our bodies manifest physically what we have been feeling emotionally and what we have been processing mentally. We feel and think about what our bodies then give us feedback on. Our mental, emotional, and physical health is interwoven and cannot be disconnected. They affect each other and have equal importance to our well-being and impact every aspect of our lives, including our businesses and careers. When we try to operate in environments that do not support all three elements of what we are, there are dangerous, potentially devastating implications, and that takes a lot of effort to undo.

What I learned was that we are not designed to work hard. Sure, we can do it for short stints of time, but remember that even then your well-being is suffering, and you will require time and extra effort to recover afterward. One sleep-in sadly just won't cut it.

We require movement, (whether that is solo or something done with assistance). In fact, we often think better and feel better when we are moving. Our chemical and hormonal supply and the timing of their release, the inflammation in our bodies and resulting pain, our immune system function, our digestive function (eating, absorbing nutrients, pooping, urinating, detoxing, etc.), the strength of our bones, our balance, and our ability to think clearly are all affected by movement. You need to exercise. You also need to rest, which can include or be done through play.

We are designed to think and feel. We produce tears for a reason. Our bodies absorb what we think and feel quite literally with the impact of what's happening in our minds, making its way down to our cellular level. What we think and feel can prime our bodies for a more positive or more negative experience of life and well-being one cell at a time. The thoughts we allow to rule our lives and the emotions we choose to express proactively versus the ones we choose to swallow determine so much more than you likely realize.

To simplify, what we think and feel affects the messages, or transmissions, sent out across our body. The body receives them and sends transmissions back to the brain, where they are interpreted for us. We cannot separate any of it because *it isn't designed to be separate.* We evolved to be the most powerful species on the planet, from our interwoven nature, which is what defines us as unique in so many ways. It's a privilege to be born into something this special, and we aren't using it!

When I recognized that the key to being successful and making that success sustainable was to tap into my humanness and let go of the false idea of working hard as being a pathway to where I wanted to go, I started to restructure my life. When I launched my business, I applied it there too. There was no way I was going to launch my business only to fall into a burnout pattern again!

For me, in both business and life, the aim of the game is to be human, and I mean HUMAN. It is the gateway to everything I think and take action on. It is the lens through which I observe my life. It is the measure of my success. If something seems unachievable without sacrificing my humanness to get there, then I don't do it. I want success to mean having the ability to enjoy and sustain it. If I can't do it healthily, I will not attempt it, because there is no point. Anything that threatens my humanness will simply be manifested by my body or mind and rear its ugly head later, so I have waved a long goodbye to letting myself do that. I let myself play, rest, move, feel, and release.

I have nonnegotiables in life now, and as a result in business. Human is my total operating system. Every single day, no matter what else I have on, taking action on my mental, physical, and emotional health is on the agenda. It doesn't matter if I am stepping off a plane, designing a new fitness system, or recording a podcast. You can bet I have also made time for all three aspects of my health. And I bring that into how I operate as a leader. I don't fall into the many traps I have spotted: I don't triple book myself for meetings, I don't work over lunch, I don't ignore what I need. My daytime schedule may be a meeting followed by a stretch, followed by a call, followed by meditation, and so on. I bring my full human to work with me. I do not relegate it to after five p.m. only. This does not waste my time; this enhances it dramatically.

This has worked so effectively for me that I recognize that I am a much better leader now than I ever would have been had I just worked hard. When I allow myself to embrace and use my full humanness, I am leading by example. I am showing my team that they have a right to be human and to be healthy. I am purposefully normalizing humanness in the way I lead. I bring wellness into the workplace, using breathing techniques to shorten meeting times by upping cognitive function and productivity, for example. I take business calls when I am actively walking or moving, where permitted, because I know that it affects my processing power, and any stress I am feeling on the call ends up being walked out rather than manifesting in my body. I knew that in the community I built, if I set this example, it would be mirrored by those who come into contact with me or the services and products I provide. I am showing you that you can achieve your goals and not be a stressed-out mess as a result. Being human has allowed me to be more empathetic and to craft my business to help my team grow in ways that work for them too. I make much better decisions, which saves me time and money since I don't have to fix as many mistakes. I am way more productive in a lot less time, which is great since I really do not want a seven-days-a-week traditional business. And I have purposefully built my business to have many systems so that when I am out for the count, my business can operate without me for stretches of time. All of this has come from ensuring that my humanness is at the top of the agenda, not the bottom of it. I have achieved more in a few years of business without getting close to burnout than I ever did by "working hard."

So regardless of whether you are studying, you are a parent, you have a business or a job, or you are just trying to get through the day, let me lay out what I think you should know. You can't make good decisions with an unrested, overstimulated mind and body. You cannot possibly be a good listener or get the most out of your days on this earth if you are tired, sluggish, or feeling crappy because you don't make time to love or move your body, eat well, drink some water, rest, or have an awareness of what you are consuming with your mind. You can't be the best caregiver in the world if your tank is always empty. You cannot create a thriving environment at home for your family or in the office when you are the living example of bottled-up stress. **You cannot lead others without first leading yourself.**

Your team, your kids, and your partners will mirror you without even thinking about it because mirroring is a way we learn from the day we are born to the day we die. We do it all the time. You will affect the well-being of everyone around you. Intense? Yes. It's a lot of responsibility, and that's why the focus has to be steered away from "working hard" to being human, which I believe is the definition of *working smart*.

My one job, really, as a CEO, a wife, a family member, or a friend, is to just be the best human I can be. I can't be the best at anything or get the most enjoyment out of this privilege that is life without being the best human I can be. That's truly it. When I respect and act on my mental, emotional, and physical health with no room for negotiation, then my potential has no limit. Human beings are capable of so much when we let ourselves actually be what we are.

Whatever it is you are looking for or wanting to achieve comes from your willingness to recognize, respect, and act on your humanness. So just be a human already!

WELLNESS TIP:
Your Human Checklist

Being the best leader, parent, friend, partner, employee, et cetera will only happen in a way you can sustain if you are taking care of your basic human needs. You may not be able to do it all at once, and it will take time to get used to checking the boxes. Start small by tackling one mini piece at a time until you have found what works for you and are doing it in sustainable ways. To ensure that I address the physical, mental, and emotional, I build it into my workday, and it is 100 percent nonnegotiable. I will do a breathing technique before a meeting, block out two minutes to stretch, meditate in the afternoon for three to five minutes, and so on. Not everything has to be done in huge blocks of time. Make it work for you in a way you can manage, and build it up over a period of months till it becomes second nature. It seems like a lot, but you will get more done in less time once this is established.

Physical health: Have I exercised (moved my body with or without assistance in some way), eaten something nutritious, drunk some water, rested, and sought out professional assistance from a doctor, naturopath, nutritionist, or osteopath (if needed)?

Mental health: Am I manually addressing my thought patterns (self-talk, mantra, taking note of my negative and positive triggers), or considering what music, shows, and texts I allow myself to consume?

Emotional health: Have I expressed myself (to a trusted party if needed), or participated in acts of mindfulness (meditation, breathing techniques, gratitude journal, etc.)?

10

EMBRACE LEVITY

I'm not kidding when I claim that I scored the greatest family in the world. They are the most supportive bunch of people who have watched, guided me, and cheered me on in everything I've ever attempted, including the things that probably worried them to their cores. My granny was and still remains one of my greatest heroes and inspirations—the perfect combination of generous love, support, and affection balanced with an open-minded and brilliant sense of humor that, from my experience, can be rare in grandparents. Grannykins (as she was known to the family) was a lot like Betty White: smart, wickedly funny, and genuinely kind. I was lucky enough to spend lots of quality time with her growing up.

Throughout my childhood, I was aware that there had been some challenging moments in her life, but we didn't really delve into the details. However, from what I did know, her energy and enthusiasm for life and for her family were gifts because she could have easily become bitter, cold, and angry instead. When I was old enough, she told me more about her story. It's not mine to tell, Gran was very private, and I will honor that; but it made me love and admire her even more. I will say this: Gran faced extreme adversity and yet lived her life with grace and levity, the kind that is only earned by going head-to-head with personal demons and making a choice to rise above it all. What a role model! I carry her with me every day.

My point isn't to tease you with details of her life that I won't reveal. My point is to highlight why any advice I got from her throughout my life was extra special. Her advice was worth its weight in gold. In fact, I could probably pen a book called "Advice from My Gran" as I have used so much of it in my own journey. But out of all the amazing wisdom she imparted upon me, one bit, in particular, has meant the most to me, and I want to share it with you.

Anytime Gran made a mistake, or something went a little pear-shaped, she'd look at me, smile, and say, "If you can't laugh at yourself, what's the point?" She'd have a laugh and get on with it or have a chat and a giggle about whatever had happened. As a kid, I could conceptualize the importance of this statement paired with seemingly trivial things, like accidentally breaking a dinner plate or forgetting to go to a scheduled appointment. And this same sense of levity was clearly passed down to my dad, who has often laughed in the face of life's quirks. But it took me a really long time to truly *get it* in the way I believe she intended it.

So many things come up in conversation when you have a stigmatized condition that feel deeply hurtful and personal, just by chance. For example, I battle with my weight sometimes, not to lose it but to gain and maintain it, especially after having a flare-up. In attempts to be open and honest in my journey, there have been times I have joined in on conversations about our experiences with our bodies. When I have opened up and shared my truth and my concerns about the impact of my weight loss on my well-being, I have been treated poorly. Rapid weight loss is very dangerous and leaves people like me with no "buffer," which protects the body against infection or allows them the resources to function day to day. In fact, my menstrual cycle has shut down completely many times because of the loss of weight. It has a huge impact on the body and is a scary position to be in. But in response to my statements, I would be told, "I wish I had your disease then. I don't know what you're complaining about," or "You can't say stuff like that. Some of us are really struggling with our weight and wish we could be skinny like you."

On the flip side, if I had been taking steroid-based medications, for example, I would sometimes look puffy, my skin would be red and unhealthy, and I would have breakouts on my face. My hair would become dry and wiry, and I would retain water. In those time periods, I would be told, "You look awful. Why aren't you looking after yourself better?" "Put on some makeup please," or "Why do you look so puffy?"

Needless to say, these are the kinds of interactions that keep invisible illness invisible. Those of us suffering in silence stay silent because we are judged or told that our experiences are invalid compared to the everyday person's. This leads to a whole range of body-image issues and mental health issues that just add to the already complex nature of what we face. It's a slippery slope.

I had decided overall that it was too stressful, to be honest, so I would simply act OK instead. I became accustomed to acting through pain and mental anguish. My husband, being the amazing soul he is, is one of the only people who can see through any façade I have used to function in the world. He's my biggest blessing.

A few years ago, the only way I could imagine being able to live my life was to get through it silently without being labeled as a victim, "a whinger," as weak or as "the sick girl." As a result, I was very embarrassed and ashamed of having a disease, particularly if it became obvious to someone else that I had one. The fear of being "caught out" was toxic, and I couldn't find any humor in my situation. My life was very serious.

In the couple of decades since I started this whole journey, I had worked out the links between my mind and body. I'd observed that anything I bottled up mentally or emotionally would present itself in my body, making any pain I experienced ten times worse, and often undermining my immune system too. The more silent I was about my truth, the sicker I actually became. But the more I talked about it and received negative feedback, the more I felt obliged to stay in the dark. It was a bad cycle to be stuck in. It occurred to me only a handful of years ago that the world was not going to change to fit me. I was going to have to create my own version of the world to live in.

So I started to live my truth and my humanness more openly little by little, starting with those closest to me, and as I gained confidence, I started to share it with colleagues and acquaintances. I still face some of the issues I faced then. Society still doesn't understand invisible illness, and certainly not Crohn's and the true lived experience of it. To make matters worse, it's easy to convince oneself that society also has little desire to learn about it. All progress takes significant time and a willingness to voice the unspoken. I started to be that voice. It wasn't altruistic. It really was for me initially. I was just so sick of fighting what I am in my entirety in order to pacify others or make them feel more comfortable with their own lives. I figured if someone wanted to dish it out, I was strong enough to take it if it meant that I ended up having one less person to act OK in front of.

A few years ago, I had a beautician appointment scheduled for my routine waxing. As I made my way to the clinic, I could feel pressure in my abdomen, and as I was walking, I could feel my belly pressing against the zipper of my pants. I was swelling up, and fast. By the time I checked in for my appointment, I looked about eight months pregnant and had broken out into a charming flop sweat. I was nauseated and incredibly uncomfortable.

I'd been going to this beautician for a while, but I had never told her about my health. I had even dodged a few questions about scars, weight loss, my hair condition, and the breakouts on my skin. I played all of it off as no big deal. I was too ashamed to admit what I had. But on this day, I knew she would ask questions, given I was so much larger than I usually looked.

I got all set up in the treatment room, removing my pants and underwear, lying back on the table, and placing a towel over my privates and big gut. I'd booked in for a Brazilian, among other things. I knew the appointment was about to get interesting!

My beautician entered the treatment room, took one look at me, and said, "Did you get very pregnant between last month and this month? What's going on?"

"No, it's nothing. So do you think it's worth me tinting my eyebrows this time?" I responded, steering the conversation away from the obvious.

I felt really embarrassed and tried to pretend that everything was OK, but I was feeling progressively worse as I lay there. My hands were dripping with sweat, and I was trying my best to control the waves of pain as my stomach expanded beyond my normal skin elasticity. It really does hurt a hell of a lot when this happens.

We managed to get through the leg and eyebrow waxing unscathed, and I knew it was time to get the privates out. As my beautician prepared the hot wax and fabric strips used for pulling the wax off the skin, I could feel the intensity in my intestines taking hold and the spasms kicking in. It felt like my insides were twisting and rotating and changing positions. Having experienced this many times, I knew I was not in any danger and that eventually this would die down to a manageable level. I just had to get through it till then and keep my fingers crossed that vomiting or diarrhea wasn't in the cards, especially as I had no pants on!

Sometimes when my intestines spasm, there's a lot of gas and fermentation and, of course, waste that is moving about. It gets caught in pockets, and the spasms sort of force it into different places as it looks for a way to exit or for the gas to dissipate—a little like making a balloon animal. I could feel everything starting to move around rapidly, and there was nothing I could do about it.

As the beautician pulled the towel off my gut and private areas to wax me, she was clearly struck by what she saw, as she audibly gasped and put her hand over her mouth in shock. Just as she began to do her job, my gut started to make the most terrifying series of growls, rumbles, bubbles, and pops. As the gas and the contents in my colon moved about with each spasm, it was visible under my taught skin, a little like when a baby's foot protrudes from its mum's tummy when it kicks. The only difference is that, instead of a foot, my protrusion looked like snakes inside of me, moving about and looking to burst their way out. Combined with the sound, it looked like I was playing host to something that was very alive, very angry, and desperate for its freedom.

I looked up at her shocked face and down at my gut and sweaty skin, realizing that what she was seeing must have looked like the scene in the film *Alien* where the alien bursts out of the stomach of a human. It really looked disturbing. I was mortified for a moment, and that's the exact second that my gran's advice came into my mind. I finally understood what to do. At that moment, all of my shock and embarrassment dropped away. I had nothing to be ashamed of or embarrassed about. It's not like I chose this. So I laughed!

I looked up at my deeply concerned beautician, and between giggles, I explained to her what was going on and why. I told her that I understood her shock but that she needn't walk on eggshells because of it. I explained that this was just part of my life, and I just wanted to be treated like she would anyone else. I encouraged her to join me in a giggle, and we broke the tension, both commenting on how bizarre the situation was. Once the tension had been lifted and I owned my situation, we had a great and very easy flow of conversation about invisible illness, and Crohn's in particular. She'd never heard of either (which is not uncommon), and she had lots of intelligent questions to ask. I happily answered them, and as we had this dialogue, she got on with her job. That moment changed our relationship from client and service provider to human and human. It was an enlightening and uplifting experience for us both.

I remained her client for quite some time till she moved away, and in subsequent treatments, she always made a point of kindly checking on my well-being without ever once making me feel like a victim, as if I needed to be wrapped up in cotton wool like I was weak or damaged.

She made me feel seen and ultimately like just a human. We even joked about my stomach "alien" a few times.

My gran's advice worked on many levels. First of all, having a laugh at your own situation can be freeing and can make you feel much better because the act of laughing helps the body release endorphins. So the tough moments don't always have to be so serious and dark. That situation was strange for the beautician and me, and either we could have made it awkward and unbearable or I could take ownership and acknowledge the absurdity of it and let the pressure out of the room by granting us both permission to smile through it. I chose to smile.

Secondly, I was able to use the situation to better my personal experience—one less person to act OK in front of. What a relief! Thirdly, this actually inspired her to have a conversation with her own family about invisible illness and Crohn's disease because she wanted them not to perpetuate any stigma that existed in the world, which I had told her about. Gran's advice helped me to facilitate the breaking down of barriers between myself and someone with no lived experience like my own. And this is how change really happens: from one person to the next and to the next and so on. There is no special switch to make everyone learn or change their behavior. It's connection and time that gets us there.

In the literal sense, I did actually laugh at myself. But I think the deeper lesson built into Gran's wise words was that we all ultimately have the choice to take ownership of our vulnerabilities, or we can let the world own them. I still think about this when I am facing off against things that pop up in other areas of life. It's applicable everywhere.

Like many of you, I had always perceived my vulnerabilities as weaknesses. I now think of them as my strengths and the source of my power and value. But I had to take ownership of them for my mindset to change.

On that day getting waxed, I was incredibly vulnerable. I tried to hide it, but on that occasion, I really couldn't get away with it. By owning my vulnerability, I cemented an idea that hasn't left me since: it is through our ownership of our personal vulnerabilities that we make true human connections and create pathways for change and growth. The world didn't become a kinder place for me to reside in by hiding all that I am or by allowing my mind to make every bad moment into a devastating blow. My life experience wasn't getting better by swallowing down shame and fear and embarrassment. It was absolutely toxic to my health to keep repeating things that didn't work for me, even if it made the people around me more comfortable.

Vulnerability was the key to the door that had the potential to open up to the rest of my life. Everything I wanted and needed was on the other side of that door: true support, the chance to positively impact others through my authenticity, and the ability to live as myself instead of faking it. I realized that if I could just live my life openly, then I might be able to get a few more people to start conversations about invisible illness, like my beautician had felt inspired to do with her own family. I knew that the more often these conversations and human connections occurred, the greater the chance that people being born with conditions like mine would not have to face as much silent suffering in their own lives.

In business, career, relationships with our significant others, and, yes, even at the monthly waxing appointment, you and I will continue to be faced with our vulnerabilities. You can't avoid them forever. What a waste of time and precious energy it is to pretend. How sad is it that we put pressure on our hard-working bodies and minds to silently absorb our issues so we can appease others? *The real shame is never in what we face personally; it is in what we allow to dictate our quality of life.*

This whole beautiful, messy experience need not be wasted trying to achieve someone else's palatable version of existence. Instead, let's be present in the absurdity of it. Some of the human experience is laugh-out-loud accidentally-snorting-through-your-nose funny and weird. Revel in your mishaps and the things you do or experience that don't fit the norm. You're here anyway, so do the whole thing gloriously. Play loud (as the forte music symbol tattooed on my arm reminds me daily).

When we step into our vulnerability, that first moment is terrifying. But once you're there, you get to tap into your innate power as a human, your ability to connect and share understanding, to learn, to grow, and to help each other get a good experience while we have the chance to be on this planet. You hold the key to making this happen for yourself. Your power and value and strength are already there, but you need to unlock them with ownership of who you are.

Gran finished her wise words with "What's the point?" I believe she meant that we could easily make our whole lives a monumental and painful challenge. I believe she was telling me to own whatever comes my way instead of letting it bury me. I believe she meant that there is a way to get through this life with levity, choice, joy, and love even when the worst things are put in front of you. She was guiding me to face off against my obstacles without making them into drama that could steal my energy and my happiness. She was telling me to be me—all of me, even the bits I might feel obliged to hide. There is not a week that goes by that I don't think about what she told me.

So when you think your vulnerability is about to be uncovered or you spot darkness on the horizon, start thinking about your vulnerability as connection and power instead. Next time things go wrong, observe the strangeness and absurdity of the situation and ease your own tension with a laugh. Take ownership of yourself, my fellow human.

It is only fitting that Gran's wisdom could be your mantra if you'd like to try it. I know it's done wonders for me. So repeat after me six times: If you can't laugh at yourself, what's the point?

WELLNESS TIP:
Hacking Your Vagus Nerve

This is a breathing technique reportedly used by Navy SEALS to improve their cognition and maintain physical health in states of stress and sleep deprivation. I have found it to be useful in managing pain, the impact of brain fog, and periods of illness and anxiety, as well as in reducing meeting times with groups of people by reducing unproductive thoughts and unneeded tension. I also encourage parents to do these techniques with their children so they have sustainable coping strategies for life.

Why It Works
When we inhale, the beat-to-beat intervals of the heart shorten slightly. When we exhale, the parasympathetic nervous system triggers the vagus nerve via secretions of a transmitter substance (ACh), which causes the beat-to-beat intervals of the heart to increase. This allows people to control the instances where the fight-or-flight response (sympathetic nervous system) may typically be triggered, making you feel wired, stressed, and panicky.

Two Methods to Try

1. The 4:8 Method:

- Inhale through the nose for a count of four. Exhale through the mouth for a count of eight. Repeat until a feeling of gentle sinking washes over you.

2. The 4:7:4 Method:

- Inhale through the nose for a count of four. Hold your breath for a count of seven. Exhale through the mouth for a count of four. Repeat until you feel a floating or gentle sinking feeling wash over you. This method can take more practice but has deeper meditative qualities, from my experience.

Both generally take anywhere from sixty seconds to five minutes to work. The more you practice this, the easier it will become for you to activate it.

11

LOVE YOUR
SUPERCOMPUTER

"You're the most coordinated uncoordinated person I have ever met," Diesel said to me between laughs one day early on in our relationship. I was laughing too. I had just attempted to walk through a wide-open doorway and had managed to bash my hip bone into the doorframe on the way through; I did little things like that a lot. As a dancer on stage, I had become adept at using my peripheral vision to ensure I was in the right position and would not collide with other dancers. I had fantastic core strength and stability. But off stage, it was not always the same. Diesel has seen me at peak performance, when I seem unstoppable, and he's also seen me in my "out of it" wobbly moments, when even getting through an open door can seem like a challenge. I have always found these phases to be quite amusing and passed them off as some kind of innate clumsiness or forgetfulness. People have quirks, and I figured this was just one of mine, no big deal, really.

But along the way, with a greater awareness of my body and health as I continued traveling down the wellness path, I began to draw a connection between these vague and wobbly moments and the experience of pain or periods of illness. Feeling as though I had mastered the other areas of my health and well-being, for the most part, I decided it might be worth thinking about whether my brain was malfunctioning or if this bashing-into-doorframes-style behavior was just part of my nature. I figured that if it turned out that I did have a brain issue, it was better to know about it and see if I could change it myself, like I had adjusted so many other things.

For example, it made sense to me that I would be groggy, moody, and less productive in the days that followed a bad night of pain or illness. The fluctuation in my hormones being regulated by my endocrine system would certainly be out of whack because of having less sleep. Sleep deprivation can cause all sorts of issues within the brain and body, let alone what pain can do. But I had a gut feeling that this was about more than a lack of sleep.

One morning, in particular, I was trying to get ready for the day ahead but was really struggling to get my normal morning routine done. During breakfast, I kept walking to the fridge, completely convinced that I was doing this for a reason, but I was unable to remember what the reason was. I would open the fridge and look in it, hoping to find the answer, and when it wouldn't come, I would close the fridge and walk away, shaking my head. I could practically see what I was trying to do in my mind's eye, but it was just slightly out of my reach. I was circling the fridge like a dog chasing its own tail, and I must have done this loop ten or more times before I threw in the towel and decided to let it go. But it bugged me because I could *feel* that I was so close to the answer, yet it just wouldn't come to me.

Throughout the next thirty minutes, I struggled to concentrate and follow my thoughts through to their natural end. I would go to write something down, only to lose half the words of the sentence, or write one that made no sense at all. I kept on losing physical items like my phone, my pen, and my lipstick. It felt like these things had just grown legs, got up, and walked out of my apartment. And if anything could be bumped into, tripped over, or dropped, I was doing it! It was frustrating, and although I didn't feel distraught about it, I was starting to feel a little moody and anxious. I just wanted to eat my breakfast and get on with my day!

I didn't forget big things, thankfully, like how to do my work or eat at the right times. It was just all these little things that accumulated to a lot of unproductive, emotional time. And the emotion could trigger that sense of distrust I had with myself, courtesy of my PTSD from my early years. Nonetheless, I continued on with my day and passed it off with a shrug. Stuff happens.

Later in the day, I went to make myself a sandwich for lunch, and when I went to the fridge to retrieve the dairy-free spread I use, it was missing. But inside the fridge, I found my phone, "lost" for hours, happily chilling on the second shelf, and right next to it was my facial cleanser. I laughed out loud. *OK, that's weird*, I thought. I grabbed my cold phone and put it on the coffee table where I could see it and carried my cleanser into the bathroom to return it to the shower, where I normally kept it. And that's where I found the nondairy spread. Sitting on the floor of the shower, now nicely melted, and my lipstick sitting next to it. "OK, that's not right at all," I mumbled to myself as I started putting things back in their rightful homes.

We all have what I like to call "brain farts" from time to time, but this was more than a fart, and this was not the first time I had discovered these kinds of things. These little things would happen quite often when I was in high levels of pain or if I had been sick for some time. In fact, I can honestly say I have done these things since Crohn's first came into my life, but I had always passed them off as silly things I did and nothing more. But I couldn't forget what I had now seen, and I was hyperaware that I was doing this with some regularity. Diesel had mentioned on numerous occasions that I would get quite vague and drift away in my mind during conversations, forgetting to respond to questions along with my train of thought, or that I would get a bit panicky if I was asked a question and couldn't seem to find the answer. I would also become very sensitive and take on a different personality when I was really under the weather, and later forget that I had said or done things amid the fog. He has always been very understanding and accepting of these things. But I placed the two pieces together and decided that the vagueness, emotional and behavioral changes, and the forgetfulness and clumsiness could all be related to Crohn's and, in particular, to the brain.

So I began researching with enthusiasm. After more than a decade of living with an invisible illness, I had never once been told about brain issues related to my condition. Then again, no one had told me about the mental health impacts, the joint and muscle pains, and a hundred other things. I was well aware that there was a gulf of missed information between the lived experience of what I had and what physicians sometimes told those of us with the condition, or even knew about it. I concluded that this could be in that same gulf of mystery. **Just because you haven't been told about it doesn't mean it doesn't exist!**

I got out Dr. Google and started tapping away at the keyboard. Loads of research papers and articles and forums started popping up. I read and read and read and read. There was so much evidence that supported a link between cognitive function, emotional change, behavioral change, memory issues, and chronic pain and illness. I could immediately reconcile a lot of it, as I used my understanding of chemical manipulation in the brain and body daily to cope with pain. I intrinsically understood that being in pain meant chemicals were firing with a regularity that other people didn't have, causing emotional change and much more. And I knew my brain would be highly fatigued as my neurons fired constantly due to my pain-perception and risk-assessment areas being on all the time; largely the amygdala, but also multiple other sectors of the brain are on because they receive and then interpret pain messages from the body. I was dismayed, though, to find so many people just like me on these forums asking the same questions. Sadly, most of them concluded that they were "nuts," "stupid," or "weak" because they'd been told that these vague, forgetful, emotional moments were not real or valid.

Much researching later, I stumbled across the term *brain fog* in relation to inflammatory bowel diseases and a variety of autoimmune diseases. All of the material listed ticked the boxes for me of what I had been experiencing. What I discovered but had never been told was that, during an episode of brain fog, the cognitive function of someone like myself could be up to 10 percent slower than people without brain fog. Some research even noted that brain fog can be more impairing than driving drunk. *Huzzah*, I thought. I had the base information, and I felt a little relieved. I wasn't alone in this at all. Brain fog is still being researched, and it's an area that many physicians do not or will not acknowledge. I have had doctors in emergency rooms laugh when I have told them I had been experiencing it. Only recently have I spoken to gastroenterologists and researchers who are now acknowledging that it exists and is a common issue raised by their patients.

Working alongside my full medical team, we collectively could understand that brain fog was happening anecdotally. If the body is firing chemicals in irregular ways with inflammation present, the immune system is fighting hard, and you can't absorb nutrients from your food, the body is going to show the impact in various ways. For me, one of them seems to be that my brain slows down and struggles to move things from short- to long-term memory and some of my general spatial awareness goes bye-bye.

Now satisfied that I had an umbrella term for what was going on, I decided it was time to start using myself as a guinea pig again. My aim was not to eradicate brain fog in its entirety—I always aim to accept my symptoms and then understand them, as this is simply kinder to myself—my aim was to make as much of my life as awesome as possible. I had been able to do this with other parts of my life through movement, food, and mindfulness, so, as far as I was concerned, the brain should be treated the same way. Without knowing it yet, I had been actively creating new pathways for default responses to pain and illness for years. My experience of pain, like everyone's, is really a sequence of neural firings, and I had been manipulating that understanding to my benefit for a long time. So I put my metaphorical boxing gloves on and got into the ring. I, the reigning featherweight, was about to do battle with the reigning heavyweight, my brain. I was ready to rumble.

I studied, experimented, and hypothesized all sorts of things. I got in the ring and threw punches that never quite landed. But as I kept going, I swung some punches that made contact! I found that on my bad pain and brain fog days, the speed with which I responded to it with movement was key to its reduced impact. I had worked out that I could up my endorphins and serotonin, reduce adrenaline, and release oxytocin if I moved my body in flow combined with mindful breathing, especially vagus nerve breathing, which numbed a certain amount of the pain, effectively bringing it within the realm of my control. This then allowed my brain to have less to worry about. Therefore, I was not draining my brain's limited resources. But there were times it might take me an hour or more to summon the will to do it. I started practicing the art of just doing it and not waiting. Adjusting those chemicals and reducing the inflammation quickly is key, largely because it stops my sympathetic nervous system (fight-or-flight response) from taking over, which disables the immune system and various other bodily functions while increasing my heart rate and emotional responses. The first five minutes always feel like I am trying to climb a mountain, but when the chemicals change and I activate the part of the brain responsible for sentimental memory through dance-like movement and music, I am golden! In fact, even my clumsiness and productivity improve!

Certain types of movements, like dancing and some forms of yoga, tap into areas of the brain related to emotion, increasing neural activity, adjusting chemical and pain response in a way that doesn't occur with other styles of movement. It works a treat for chronic pain, which is why it's fundamental in my own Corethentic system.

I also worked out that putting nutrient-dense, anti-inflammatory fuels into my body when I was ill or in pain also affected my brain. I keep a supply of bone broth (amazing for the immune system and easily absorbed by the gut), thyme to make thyme tea (expectorant and detox properties, bloat reduction, inflammation response), sweet potato (dietary fiber, inflammation response, energy) and electrolyte popsicles on hand because what I put in does help determine what I get out. I make my brain's and body's jobs as easy as I humanly can, as then it makes my life easier too.

I upped my use of mindfulness techniques like meditation, mantra, and gratitude, making them entirely nonnegotiable parts of how I operate because they help to adjust my chemicals and hormones, and prime the brain and body for positivity instead of negativity. These things are on my calendar, even during a busy day. These can be used in practically any circumstance for pain reduction and emotional control. It is a convenient way to get relief! I keep on telling my brain and body what I want from them. I do the work; they facilitate.

On pain days, I went from around 10 percent cognitive impairment to 5–6 percent when I am in pain for many days or weeks, and only 3–4 percent when I am in pain on a single day. There are variables, but my average day-to-day impairment is much lower than it was before! But, as always, I learned something wider reaching than I had expected from all of this. My brain could be positively manipulated. So that means that the average person could do it too. Surely we all have untapped potential we know nothing about that could make our lives better if we had a way to use it!

I started to think about the brain in general. I had been teaching my clients for years that exercise was just "brain training for the body." I knew that the brain was undergoing a huge process of creating neural links inside itself and then sending off signals to nerves and muscles to do things they sometimes had never been asked to do before. The brain is a very busy machine doing work in the background every second of the day and night. Asking it to do anything new means it's going to have to work on it for a while and fit it into its busy schedule, using limited resources to make it happen. I wanted my clients to understand that it was going to take time to see the physical manifestation of the work their brain was doing. It will never, ever be immediate. But I started to think this idea might also be applicable to what we think, especially when we are hurting in one way or another.

We brain train ourselves all the time! Not just when we are kids. We are doing it throughout life. Taking a different route home from work and wanting to remember it is brain training. Styling your hair differently is brain training. Remembering to make the bed in the morning is brain training. Quite literally anything you think, do, or act on is brain training. None of it just "shows up" by chance. We don't spend much time looking at the process of how things came to be in our lives. We just focus on the end result. This is what leads us to think, *I just do that*, or *I can't do that.*

The brain is all about efficiency once it has locked something down. It's too busy to start from scratch every time. Its job is not to decide for you what inner dialogue is going to be good versus bad for you. Its job is to keep you alive as efficiently as it can. So if you keep saying, "I am silly," over and over again, guess what you end up believing? The brain simply knows you have told it to create a system of transmissions around that, and because you keep repeating it, it interprets that to mean, "This seems like something you will keep triggering, and I am busy, so I am going to connect all this up so when you are triggered to think about this, I will just take you straight to it to save time." It is a powerful tool and very easy to use for our own self-destruction! In my case, I became curious about how I could make it constructive instead.

That's when I became obsessed with the brain and wanted to understand why some of the things I was doing seemed to work and what things were not working at all. I wanted to know how I could extrapolate that to help others. I studied and earned my diploma of neuroplasticity. Neuroplasticity is used in various ways by different types of professionals like psychologists and researchers, for example, but is primarily the term that describes a wide range of phenomena around brain adaption, change, and processing. To me, it takes the saying "You can't teach old dogs new tricks" and throws it right out the window!

I'd long been a fan of mantra and meditation, using them to keep myself focused and positive, especially during flare-ups. However, they also allowed me to be more adaptive, cope better with change, and accelerate my own progress. If you have ever had a brilliant idea and then forgot it before you had a chance to explain what it was, it is because you didn't give the brain the reinforcement needed to turn that spark into a neuron, and eventually a neural pathway. We have to build neural pathways (neurons connected by dendrites) for ideas to stick. Then our brain cells start to "chat" to each other, which is called *neural firing*.

So anything I now want to work on, think about, change, or achieve is something I reinforce with immediacy and enthusiasm. I always come back to "this is just brain training" and set to work, creating as many dendrites as I can so that the chatter between my brain cells can begin. When I reinforce the idea with action, using as many areas of the brain at once as possible, I am creating "stickiness," or linking between more regions of the brain and the idea. This means I can start creating new default pathways for the brain, replacing the ones that are not working that well for me. So, to simplify, if I know that my brain saying, "This pain sucks and my life is so crappy," is not a helpful response to being in pain regularly, then I have the power to get my brain to respond to that pain with "OK, we have done this before; let's start using some of our tools to make this a bit better," instead. I am sure you will agree that the latter is a healthier response!

When I am in pain, I try not to pile onto myself using my old neural pathways of "Life is crap. This sucks. I hate my body." Instead, when I am in pain, my first response is "OK, let's get you up and moving so we can change those chemicals and have a good day." This is not a coincidence. This was me brain training that into my life. I stopped reinforcing a behavior that made me feel worse and replaced it with one that makes me feel better. Even separately, I have applied this to myself with wanting to learn new skills, improve my self-esteem and confidence, earn more qualifications, and so on. It all starts in the brain.

I learned that the brain does "pruning" every couple of months or so, where it lets things that are no longer reinforced drop away. This is not a bad thing but a good thing. Our super-efficient system recognizes that it has limited resources and only applies them to the things we demonstrate to it that they are important to us. I think that is a pretty impressive system!

If we keep saying negative things about ourselves, it will keep those. If we stop going for a walk every day for a while, it will decide that it wasn't super important to us and won't help us to get it done. On the plus side, this means we can train the brain to focus on new and better things. Now, not everything goes away. For example, an actual trauma is complex, but we can change the way we respond to the trauma when triggered by providing new default pathways for the brain to take.

When I want to address something and create a new pathway, I build it into as much of my life as possible so I give my brain no choice but to build that neural pathway! Different areas of the brain are responsible for different senses and responses. To speed up the process of creating a more efficient and kinder pathway for the brain to take when triggered, I ensure that when I am learning something important I have as many of my senses as possible and both hemispheres of the brain switched on. So using mantra as a prime example, I purposefully say it to myself out loud. This is because I want my auditory system switched on. It also makes a big difference for your brain to hear your voice saying something versus someone else saying it; different emotional responses may light up. I will also stand in front of the mirror when I say my mantra so that the occipital area of my brain is paying attention. I will also write the mantra down because then I am ensuring my left hemisphere is paying attention. I also learned that it takes a minimum of six repetitions to get the brain to realize we want it to remember what we are saying or doing. This then made me realize how much of our learning is learning by association as well. It brought me back to my choreography days when I would get my performers to face different directions in the room from time to time to run a rehearsal. This was because if you have only ever practiced said routine facing one side of the room, and then when you have to perform it, you are actually facing the other side, you may forget the steps! The brain is taking in oodles of information all the time that we are unaware of. When we have an experience that changes us, or we learn something vital, the brain takes almost a bird's-eye-view snapshot of our entire surroundings, which may include the temperature, furniture in the room, what we are wearing, what we can smell, see, feel, and more. This is why we have so many "triggers." Our triggers are derived partially from our associated learned memory.

So if I wanted to be able to reduce my brain fog, reduce my pain, manage my mental health, and start replacing that old, tired, toxic language I had been using on myself for many years, I was going to have to create the right conditions to do so. This is why I do my mantra everywhere I go. I will do it in a public bathroom in front of the mirror, not just the one in my home, for example. I want my brain to know that a new pathway of thinking is important to me anywhere that I am, not just in the safety of my home. And I will also do it alongside a breathing technique or meditation, as I want my body to learn these new pathways, knowing I am as calm and safe as I can be. When I am triggered to use these pathways I create, my brain will retrieve the associated memory information around it too. The brain knows whether I associate that pathway with good or bad emotions and will adjust itself accordingly. So the calmer and happier I am when I learn something new, and therefore the more serotonin is present, the happier and calmer I will be when I am triggered to use that exact pathway. The body ends up manifesting whatever I am thinking and the feelings associated with it. It's all connected.

I make a point in many of my public speaking appearances to teach these kinds of real-world skills to the audience live, no matter if we are in a loud, crowded space or a smaller, more intimate venue. **For anything in life to really work when it comes to the brain or body, it is about sustainability.** You do not need a special shrine room to meditate in, and you do not need a quiet space to make a mantra work for you. You just need to bring it with you and use it regularly; the brain will understand and adapt. This makes it more likely that the brain will respond to triggers of pain, both physical and emotional, by saying, "Maybe we should meditate now," or "Let's say our mantra six times," instead of "This sucks. I hate feeling like this."

I may never be able to undo all the damaging thoughts in my head, put there by others and reinforced so often by me over the years, all of which is deeply attached to trauma. However, what I do have the power to control is how I allow myself to respond to it now. For me, understanding that I can add better things to my brain gave me a lot of hope. I have used this understanding of myself to create much more beneficial inner chatter, which has been critical to my health overall.

Mantra, in particular, is something I practice daily alongside meditation and movement. I do it when I am in pain and when I am coping well. But on those awful days, if I get myself moving, say a mantra on repeat and meditate, or do some breathing, it is like I am rewiring my responses from the inside out. Because I am! This has reduced my brain fog, my issues with balance and spatial awareness, and my pain, and has improved my immunity, gut function, mood, sleep, and more. When I do not do these things, life is pretty brutal. So for me, it is a no-brainer to do it (pun intended.....I really do love a good pun).

Most people find they have several inner tapes in their minds that aren't very helpful or kind. So I suggest tackling them one at a time instead of all at once. Dedicate a month or two to each mantra you create. Reinforce it as much as you can. While you are busy giving the brain something to do, some of the less reinforced negative stuff starts to fade into the background.

We just have to remember that the brain will always pick the *easiest* pathway to travel when triggered. The only way to make the easy path the right one for you is for you to create it and then reinforce it again and again. **Whatever is reinforced the most wins.** Eventually it sticks and the old, not-so-good pathway it had before can be "pruned" so it is no longer the first option the brain will select from.

I have used this for my health to ensure that my days are the best they possibly can be. But it is also how I have accelerated my skills, grown my business, and found my way into opportunities that might not have been there otherwise. I actively train my brain to work with me rather than against me. I will still have some days when the butter ends up in the shower and my cleanser in the fridge. But I am now markedly better at many things than I was before I started looking into the capability of the brain.

I am excited that I have had the chance to share this with my clients and have been able to weave this understanding into the services I offer. People don't always know the extent to which I am helping them brain train themselves, but it is front and center with me and what I do at all times. I have passed on these skills to people who have used it and gone on to find their dream careers after stagnating for years. People are living better with pain than before. People are repairing damaged relationships. People are pivoting their business models with ease. All of this and more comes from brain training and using simple methods like mantra and meditation to achieve it.

Most of us live with a supercomputer on top of our shoulders we know nothing about. Our potential to help ourselves with our health and mindset; to attain more knowledge; to become more productive, kinder, more confident, or better leaders; to have greater success in business or our jobs; to be better parents; and more is ridiculous. If you know how to work with the brain to get the life you want, nothing is truly off-limits.

WELLNESS TIP:
Mantra

I encourage you to write a mantra every six to eight weeks that reflects something you would like to address, improve, or get your brain to work on. Repeat it to yourself daily a minimum of six times in a row each day. Keep it simple, to no more than two sentences, and focused on assertive language (in other words, the word *try* has no place in a mantra).

Here is one I have used before to get you started! "I am thankful for my body, as it is the only one I will ever get. So I will love her, nourish her, respect her, and allow her to evolve."

12

CRACK THE
FORMULA

Growing up both creatively and entrepreneurially minded, coupled
with everything else I had going on with my physical and mental health,
was confusing. My home life and school life were very structured and
organized, with clear routines and requirements to be met. My parents
taught me to have a strong work ethic. In my home, there was no idle
time, as there was always something to be done. I was taught I could be
anything I put my mind to. I am thankful for my acquired work ethic.
But as much as a good work ethic has been helpful for me as an adult, it
has also tied me to social expectations I have struggled to meet. I have,
at various times in my life, found it difficult to find a way to be exactly
who I am.

School was all about preparing me for the "real world," which is
great, except that I didn't really want what it had to offer, nor did I
see myself fitting into the real world. In the real world, my creativity
wasn't considered a desirable or logical pathway to pursue. In the real
world, the jobs I would be most suited for based on my natural skill
set would be harder to come by and less valued, and would mean a
smaller paycheck too. In the real world, having health issues seemed to
be deemed some kind of sin. However, in the real world, things did not
happen according to some special plan that was simple to follow, even

though we were told that it would be. In the real world, as opposed to school, there is no formula for reaching success even though we are largely all taught a universal one.

School and most of our young lives gear us to copy one another, to reach a pinnacle of success by safety. The imagined linear line goes a little like this: Get an education. Apply said education to a career path (usually picked before the age when our brains have fully developed). Stick to that career path no matter what. Eventually, buy a house and a vehicle. Go on one holiday a year. Find a mate. Procreate. Success!

I'm not here to tell you this formula is wrong. It serves many people well, and you may be one of them. If this is your version of success and you feel you have the quality of life you desire, then I genuinely congratulate you. But notice how this linear plan doesn't mention how you feel, your health, or the quality of life you live? That is because these things are highly variable from person to person, and when one wants to include these things, suddenly this linear path ends up looking a lot less linear.

Not once growing up did I find that I could reconcile what I wanted or needed from life against the formula I'd been integrated into by society. I wanted more. I wanted something different. I wanted to be in a position to use all of what came naturally and what I'd worked for *while positioning myself to be well.* To fit the formula I had been presented, I'd have to permanently shut off whole pieces of myself.

But as this was the only formula I'd been exposed to, I wasn't sure what to do. Even as I steered my ship into creative waters, and then again into health pools, I was wracked with guilt. It felt like I was failing life by doing what I was good at and what made me feel good, not ticking the boxes of everyone else's life. Even as I achieved success in my chosen fields and became a lot more functional, I felt like I was a loser in everyone else's eyes.

I am thankful and grateful every day that I met my husband and that he's wired like I am, both creative and entrepreneurial. The only traditional thing we have ever really done is to get married. Pretty much every other aspect of our lives has been an example of breaking away from the linear formula we'd both been educated into. I have someone by my side who lives his authenticity, and that's helped me to live mine. It's made me healthier too!

By being truly who I am, it's eased the pressure on my body. I do not have to be a fake version of myself to satisfy an employer. I have purposefully structured my business so that I can be at the forefront or the background to suit my body. Therefore, my stress levels are lower, which means my immunity is stronger, my pain is more manageable, and I can move with speed and accuracy towards my goals, which were out of my reach when trying to live in the predetermined straight line.

Here's what I have observed. The general formula of life we get taught is $A + B = C$. The actual world is more like $A + B = C$, except when $A + B = Z - T$. I hate to be the bearer of bad news, but there is no true formula for everyone on the planet. We all have strengths and natural skills that vary from person to person. We all have health and well-being needs that need to be met. It's not as simple as a straight line. The truth is much curvier.

What I've also seen from my clientele and lived myself is that the best way for each of us to achieve our unique version of quality of life means living our authenticity. That equates to us living through wellness. Paying attention to what moves and drives us, what kinds of people, places, and things increase versus decrease our energy are helpful guides. Ensuring we take care of the mental, emotional, and physical regularly ensures that the mind has a relationship with the body that is built on kindness and understanding instead of resentment, betrayal, and fear. Happiness and health are worth noting as markers that can guide our unique path. When we are in tune with these things, we are again at our most human selves. That's when we are healthiest, from organs to mind, most resilient, and most aware of how we fit into the world and the effect we have on the person next to us.

When we are not aligned, when we flog ourselves or feel so guilty that we force ourselves to live this false linear formula, we are more

prone to illness, mental health issues, and other life challenges. We are also more likely to project our dissatisfaction on others to justify our own choices, which in turn stunts the personal growth of the people we come into contact with. We so often get in our own way, and others', for the sake of sticking to a formula that is unrealistic.

Before I allowed myself to be wholly dedicated to living through wellness, I would keep falling back into thinking that I had to stick to the linear line throughout life even though it had never worked well for me. So I'd look at a person who seemed to have it all together and would attempt to copy their path to get where I wanted to go. I'd look at what they'd done as a straight line. *If I do X for two years, I can get the promotion and I will have achieved "success."*

As I'd walk these paths, I would feel myself dying inside. I am not exaggerating. I could feel my soul screaming, "This is not right for you!" My body would become sicker, my mental health would take a hit, and eventually I would acknowledge that what I was doing was not going to get me to the quality of life I desired. More importantly, I realized that whatever I did, and whoever I chose to do it with, would either elevate or undermine my well-being. A bad workplace, course of study, or relationship, in my opinion, is generally not worth staying in because, sometimes unbeknownst to you, your body is aware that the environment or person is toxic. And that will slowly but surely eat away at your well-being. Eventually, for most people, a toxic work environment or relationship will cause a major reaction from the body or mind, and you will be forced to leave often well after the damage is done. This damage is then carried with you into the next one.

And we do this because we think there is some special straight-line formula, some life criteria we must meet to have value. In my roles outside of dance, I have changed jobs often. This is because my body is very clear about what works for it. For those without a chronic condition, it may take years for the issues to manifest in a permanently damaging way, even though your body will be trying to tell you in a whole variety of ways throughout that time. For me, it only takes months. This is largely because stress affects the gut catastrophically. The gut is where up to 80 percent of our serotonin is made, our happy hormone. Our gut produces 70 percent of our immune cells and 100 million brain cells and can have up to four times as many cortisol (stress hormone) receptors within it as the brain; in fact, it is often referred to as "the second brain." So you know that gut instinct thing? Yeah, don't ignore it. Your body, your gut in particular, is a regular Chatty Cathy. It is constantly trying to tell you what you need to know. When I learned this, I realized I had to do all I could to avoid disrupting my special "happy and healthy" farm where all that good stuff grows. If the gut is where it is produced, then it is where it needs to be nurtured. And this is not just done through food or supplementation! This is about being true to ourselves. When we are true to ourselves, when we do what's needed to be as well as we can be, when we walk a path of our own, we reduce the interruption to our crop of cells and hormones. We want those cells to grow and flourish, not die at our own hands.

The last time that I tried to take a linear approach was when I went to start my own business. I have never done it since. I looked at what was being offered in my industry and paid close attention to who was leading in the field at the time. I studied their behavior, how they presented themselves publicly, what they said, and how they said it. I dismissed my personal strengths because they did not match those of the leaders in my field, and tried to emulate the path that had been carved by those whom I had studied.

But at every turn, I was being ignored, knocked back, or hitting brick walls. What seemed like logical steps for my peers just didn't seem to work for me. For example, it seemed that part of their success had been a beneficial partnership or collaboration with more prominent brands in the market than themselves.

However, when I'd reach out to large companies within or associated with the industry to make time for a chat or to try to collaborate together, I would get no response whatsoever. Or I would get a very blunt rejection or a generic "no thanks"-style response. I have left hundreds of phone messages that went unreturned and sent probably hundreds of emails that went nowhere. I was told repetitively that I didn't have enough social media presence to warrant his or her effort and that I "don't look like somebody in fitness."

I had something to offer, I was following the straight line laid down by others, and I was being pushed away. Was it my tattoos? Was it because I was so short? Was I speaking in a tone that was too high pitched to be taken seriously? I questioned everything I could think of and applied dozens of changes to my behavior while sticking to the linear path to try to improve the situation. I had a spreadsheet I used to track what I was doing, and the facts spoke to me loudly. I was not getting a handful of rejections. I was getting dozens and dozens of them. I was the common denominator in the equation. I was not hitting the mark.

I took stock of the situation. I felt so sure inside that what I had to offer was worth my time and effort to get it right. I was living really, really well for someone with disease and pain, and in a way, that was on the rare side. I wanted to offer what I'd learned to the world. I wanted all of my hard knocks to mean something. So I reflected on my life experiences from the time I was a child to those I was experiencing as an adult.

I noticed a pattern when I took the time to pay attention to it. Everything that had ever worked for me in my life came left of center. Nothing that brought me success in the past had been achieved by walking in a straight line. I was never "tall enough" to be a dancer, and I was "too sick" to do it too. I wasn't experienced enough to be a choreographer, and I had no applicable skills when I first got my job at VaynerMedia. I wasn't naturally "the right body type" for the fitness industry. I got to all those places by taking the path less traveled. I seized the opportunities that others would have ignored. I hustled until people had no choice but to pay attention to me. I grew communities that helped me realize my vision and theirs simultaneously. The common pattern was that I was being authentic, which means I was healthier. I was providing myself with every reason under the sun to succeed and have a genuine quality of life at the same time.

In comparison, when I was trying to walk a straight-line path, I had to suppress parts of my personality, I had to hide parts of my reality from the world. And that was undermining my efforts to be well! It was like I was taking a flamethrower to my gorgeous crop of serotonin, brain, and immune cells and therefore giving my cortisol receptors too much fuel and giving stress too much input in my life!

I recognized that when I had been studying my idols, I had failed to see what they all had in common. What they had done for themselves in reflection may have been portrayed as some logical and deeply linear line they'd followed, but it was, in fact, a squiggly path they had taken. Not one of them really followed a formula like another. The things they did didn't match the $A + B = C$ formula at all. They were in tune with the formula that worked for *them*. Each of them had learned to understand who they were, what they wanted, and made decisions that reflected that knowledge. They tapped into their human, authentic self and traveled the loopy, zigzaggy path that took them to their destination.

I realized that I had already been taste testing the nonlinear way of living. But I kept dropping it for the straight line as I felt obliged to. That's when I said a fond farewell to the good old $A + B = C$ and hello to $A - D = Z$ and its myriad variations along the way.

As soon as I started to present myself publicly as the person I actually was, flaws, strengths, and all, the needle shifted. I attracted the right kind of clients and business relationships. I discarded ideas for my business that would steer me back onto the silly straight line and instead did what made sense to me. People started to reach out to me instead of me chasing them. **Authenticity is a powerful thing if you harness it. You can use it for a lot of good in the world.**

Instead of being the woman that sheepishly tries to fit in with others, and is usually then ignored, I am the openhearted woman who appears seemingly out of thin air to offer you a "congrats" on something you have been working on, because I mean it and will build a personal relationship with you out of that exchange. I am the businessperson that rejects a deal when I feel that the team offering it is being inauthentic, because I deal in authenticity, not just on the bottom line. I am not a good employee; I am a CEO through and through because I will spot problems with your business and feel compelled to tell you about them to help you succeed. I use my logical mind and my emotional self and always will. I express myself and prioritize my well-being over all else. I am not a robot. You will always deal with a human. I don't switch it off anymore.

You might be reading this right now, wondering how this is even remotely connected to wellness. Fair point if you are. My point is, wellness is truly holistic. **It's about being all you are to get what you want.** I truly believe now that there is nothing disconnected. So yes, even a job or a business should be designed to propel and elevate not just a product or service but the people who build it. Authenticity is timeless. Authenticity is a very healthy thing. And it's made me a better friend, wife, and leader without a doubt. When it clicked into place, I threw the rulebook out the window, erasing the straight-line mentality and accepting that the squiggly topsy-turvy path is the one that's right for me. It is a reflection of my wellness, not a distraction from it.

I've seen too many people extinguish their own flames of brilliance and live mediocre lives for the sake of following the formula they'd been educated to believe was the only one available to them. I have seen countless people allow their wellness to be eroded for the sake of staying on a path that is clearly not allowing them to flourish at all. I've seen too many people get ill and struggle as a result of the toxicity that results from the misalignment in their lives between what they think they should do and what is authentic and healthy to do. A straight line in life does not mean it is going to be right for you. Being able to stick to one path forever, forsaking all others, doesn't guarantee your success, happiness, and health. But doing what actually works for you just might.

One of the most essential lessons I have learned in my life has been to see myself in my entirety and make decisions that allow me to get where I want to go based on that instead of trying to mold myself into something that I am not. If the straight line isn't working for you, please know that there is an alternative. I am proof that you can have a strange mishmash of skills and experiences and health issues and still find a way to do it. But the key is to avoid playing copycat to someone else. Sure, use someone's example as a springboard to get you on to a path, but when your gut is telling you something is off, or when your mind or body is trying to show you that it is time to ride your own path, listen to it.

It means understanding that everything *inside* of you is connected to the quality of life reflected *outside* of you. What you then put out into the world will also make its way back in. It's understanding that your health and quality of life, your relationships, business, career, family, experiences, and goals are equal parts of the package. It's taking actions that nurture all that you are instead of one little piece.

The best stories in life are full of twists and turns. Movies are boring in a straight line, songs are filled with sideways steps that lead to forward momentum, page-turning fiction is all about the unexpected twists and the convergence of many compelling storylines into one. This is what drives us, motivates us, educates us, entertains us, fills us with purpose as people. So let your life be as squiggly as it needs to be for you to be at your most human, fabulous self. Let your path honor who you are and make your story as thrilling as the ones that remind you why life is such a privilege in the first place.

My life has been weird, beautiful, hard, painful, overwhelmingly awesome, and full of emotion. By *living human*, I am able to give this abundance of love I feel to so many more people, and the process of living this way gives it back to me in spades. What initially felt like a dark force within me that was desperate to get out and wreak havoc has been transformed into a light that heals through becoming myself. My story, as hard as it has sometimes been, is one I wouldn't trade for anyone else's. It has all happened in a perfectly imperfect way, teaching me endlessly and inspiring me daily. I find myself fascinated and so curious about what we all are. I will never stop trying to understand it even more. There is just so much of our lived experience that is interesting. We are capable of extraordinary things. I went from genuine resentment towards my body to falling into a deep love and respect for it. It is my hope you will take actions towards feeling that way about your own, being curious and kind and loving to it because it is part of every experience you have ever or will ever have. Be authentic with who you are and what you need. It will make a world of difference to you in a way I cannot describe in words. It has to be experienced.

Give this life everything you have got. Allow yourself to fall and get back up, to take side streets and make U-turns. Position yourself to be able to spread your wings and take off. Give yourself permission to find every nook and cranny, every flaw and feature, every strength and weakness. No one will give you a different body, a different mind, or a different life. The world will tell you what it thinks you can't or shouldn't do. But you, you amazing person, can reach down deep inside and open all the locked doors and then walk through them and find out what you can do. There is nothing separate; there is nothing that is not beautifully linked in the most profound, wiggly, squiggly, topsy-turvy kind of way. Your path, derived from the choices you make, whatever it brings you, pain or joy, rises and falls and plateaus—all are meant to be there for you to learn from. Life is truly bittersweet. Head towards it with your lovely human arms open, hug it tightly, squeeze the juice and color out of it, and amplify it all with everything you have within you. You are privileged because there is breath in your body. You are blessed because you are human.

WELLNESS TIP:
Gratitude Practice

Gratitude is a simple way to rewire your brain and physiologically prepare you for a better experience of life, from your cells to your neurons.

I recommend starting and ending your day by identifying at least one thing you are grateful for and writing it down, telling someone about it, or thinking about it at length.

Initially you may not think there is much to be grateful for. Instead of searching for something that is outstandingly amazing, appreciate moments that are passable, OK, or simply not bad. It will take time to seek out the good that is in your world.

When these moments of gratitude are the first thoughts in your head as you start your day and the last ones in your mind before you sleep, you will be amazed at how your approach to life alters. Remember that the brain is hard-wired for risk assessment in order to survive. In order to actually live, you will need to take the time to find the good and teach your brain that your life actually has good moments in it!

EPILOGUE

I am a certified wellness coach, personal trainer, group fitness instructor, meditation guide, dance teacher, and CEO/founder, and have diplomas in neuroplasticity and holistic pain management, and I am a mindfulness practitioner, trained to practice in a range of other specialty areas within the above scope. Still, I am not a doctor, nutritionist, naturopath, or medical professional, so my story should not be used as a diagnostic tool nor a prescription. Please seek a medical and holistic team that works for you, and please keep looking if you aren't satisfied with the one you have. The perfect ones for you are out there, but you need to be proactive. I hope you will feel empowered to learn more about you and keep seeking answers to how you tick. You *are* worth it.

All physical and mental conditions sit on a spectrum, and so the symptoms I have may be different from someone else's, and my journey may look different than someone else's. None of this happened overnight. While I have been privy to many people's stories and have seen a lot of overlap between what I have experienced and what they have, there are also some stark differences too. Each of our journeys and experiences is unique because we each come with different DNA and other factors that affect us. I have been as accurate as my occasionally foggy brain and memory can allow me to be about my own journey, but there are bits that are still fuzzy and a little out of reach due to trauma and how some of what I have experienced has impaired my long-term memory. I have adjusted some details to protect the privacy of others, and simplified some of the more complex processes I have touched on. If you fall into an invisible illness category, I hope you know I believe you, understand you, and know that what you feel is 100 percent valid *no matter what anyone else may have told you.* Above all, I hope this inspires you to get curious about your skin suit.

I am critical of the medical industry because millions of us with invisible diseases are relegated to the sidelines so often by it. But that is shifting slowly, and I have met many fantastic doctors and nurses now who really do help. If you are one of them, thank you. I also now understand that medical professionals are often the most burned-out people because of the hours they are expected to work, the things they emotionally have to take on, and the pressure of the types of decisions they have to make. These people who have worked tirelessly to become professionals are often making judgement calls about our lives on the back of working twelve or more hours straight, and rarely with their own personal wellness being prioritized. I think it would make a big difference to patients if the professionals were more well themselves, and that means the entire industry has to evolve to facilitate that. It is going to take a lot of time.

This book is one tiny snippet of my story, and I have isolated it as much as possible so that I am honoring each part of my story to the best of my ability. This book would have been far too cumbersome to read with it all included, so I had to select the most key elements and the things I have struggled with the most to write about. This has been a cathartic and terrifying process to undertake, and I have relived many traumas and exorcised many demons in order to get it out. I have cried and laughed with shaky hands as this poured out of me. Knowing this is out in the wild now is both a bucket-list moment that I am beyond grateful for and an experience that makes me feel naked. I live with my heart purposefully exposed and with my vulnerability consciously laid bare, as these are gateways to my courage. So as challenging as this has been, I am so grateful for this experience. I have grown enormously in the process of getting this part of my story out. Thank you from the bottom of my heart for letting me have this chance and for reading about it. I really do hope that no matter what you face, my story helps you realize you are capable of taking on anything your heart desires. After all, I "shouldn't" have been able to live the majority of my life.

Most days of the week, I am online reading the struggles that so many people with pain and illness face in a myriad of support groups I am involved in. Between what is shared to me directly by my own clients and those I connect with online, I am at times overwhelmed by the silent suffering that is in the world. From people sharing their suicidal thoughts with me to those celebrating making it through a whole night of sleep for the first time in years, I have been privileged to see what humans are capable of working through. I am reminded every day that invisible illness is a very real battle being faced the world over by millions of people. I am reminded every day that we can flourish, often in the most trying of circumstances. I am reminded of how far I have been able to come. I am reminded that there is hope and that we can actively teach and practice it every day. I am reminded that we are more powerful together as a species than we can ever be alone, and when we remove stigma and just see human, we can do anything. I hope future generations will embrace what they are much earlier and experience even more life than the rest of us have.

I sometimes say that I am lucky to have a business and to have done the things I have done, but it isn't really luck at all. Sure, the universe has some magical timing, but it has all been about choice and perseverance and an unrelenting belief that my experience can be of use to someone else. I believe this is true for all of us. I often say that the wellness industry will reshape all systems in the coming five years to bring out the best our species has to offer. Wellness is the vehicle that will make it happen, and I am proud to be there doing my little bit.

If you came to this book for mindset, business or health reasons, or curiosity, above all, I hope that it has demonstrated that the many parts of our lives are never actually isolated. A struggle in health can be an educator for a better way to build a business. A mindset strategy for business may amplify your health.

Nothing in isolation, everything in togetherness, truly human.

ACKNOWLEDGMENTS

I would like to acknowledge my husband, Diesel, who is my soulmate and biggest supporter and has a "no BS" attitude that challenges me to be my best every day. I could write another book on how he supports me in the things I face. Not once has he complained or thought of me as weak or someone requiring coddling. No doubt, what I have gone through has altered the direction of his life immeasurably, but you would never know it. He is the most adaptable person to change I have ever met and inspires me to embrace life daily. I will never know how to thank him for the gift of love he continues to give me. Diesel, I am deeply honored to be on this journey of life with you.

I would also like to acknowledge my family, who faithfully back me every step of the way. I do not know where they have found the strength to face having a child and sister with illnesses, and the occasionally destructive missteps I have taken to find my way, but I am grateful for their strength and have drawn on it countless times. I say all the time, "I have the best family in the world," and I mean it. You are heroes to me.

To my friends, clients, amazing team (Sofia and Tammy - you absolute gems), and supporters, I can't thank you enough. Growing up invisible, I didn't have many friends and certainly even fewer who could understand what I was trying to achieve. I now feel I have that support

I sorely missed then. Thank you for that precious gift. Thank you for trusting me with your well-being and for being so open with me week in and week out about the most vulnerable parts of your life. I will continue to work to honor them. I am in constant awe of your resilience and brilliance. You inspire me constantly.

Thank you to Alicia, Dan, Jackson, and the whole team at Indigo River Publishing, who found me on the other side of the world and have given me the chance to do this. More importantly, they have inspired me to do even more. Thank you, Adrienne, for patiently working with me as I edited this book from across the globe and allowing me to find and use my voice instead of trying to craft it into someone else's. I have learned so much from each of you. I will value those gifts for the rest of my life.